SENSORY AWARENESS

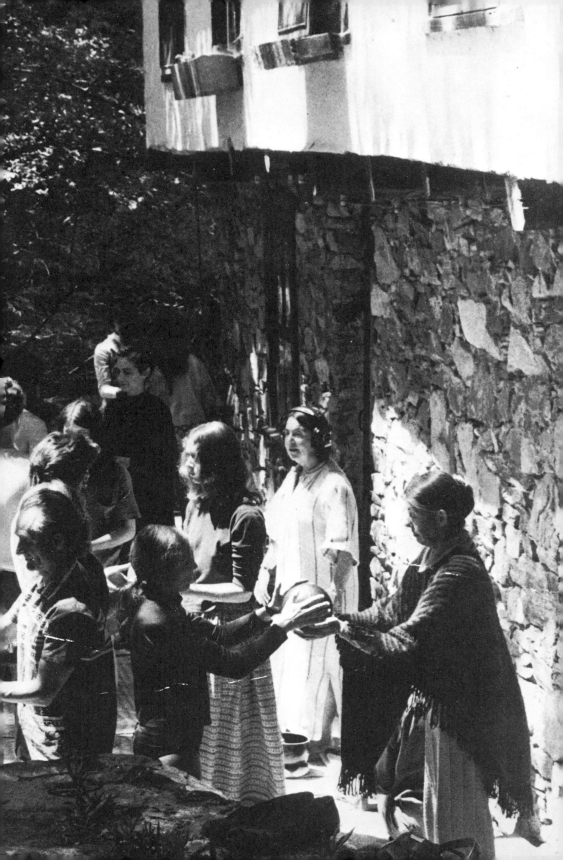

Sensory
Awareness

THE REDISCOVERY OF EXPERIENCING

CHARLES V.W. BROOKS

ROSS-ERIKSON PUBLISHERS   SANTA BARBARA

Published by Ross-Erikson, Inc., Publishers, 629 State Street, Santa Barbara, Ca. 93101

First published in 1974 by The Viking Press, Inc.

Printed in the United States of America
Library of Congress Catalog Card Number 73-7432
ISBN NO. 0-915520-56-7

All photographs in this book, except those listed below, are by the author.

PAGE xii: Alissa Goldring.   PAGES 4, 15, AND 24: Photo Mariann Reismann, from Dr. Emmi Pikler, *Que sait faire votre bébé*, Les Editeurs Français Réunis, 1951.   PAGE 27: Ansel Adams.   PAGE 48: Photo Mariann Reismann, from Dr. Emmi Pikler, *Que sait faire votre bébé*, Les Editeurs Français Réunis, 1951.   PAGES 53 AND 55: J. R. Harris, *Egyptian Art*, London: Spring Books, 1966.   PAGE 60: British Museum, London. PAGE 63: Fotocelere, Turin, Italy.   PAGE 70: Gregor Krause, *Bali: Volk, Land, Tanze*, Munich: Gregor Müller Verlag, 1926.   PAGE 71: Ylla, *Deux Petits Ours*, Guilde du Livre, Lausanne, 1954. Rapho Guillumette Pictures. PAGES 77, 78 (LEFT): Photo Mariann Reismann, from Dr. Emmi Pikler, *Que sait faire votre bébé*, Les Editeurs Français Réunis, 1951.   PAGES 80, 81: F. Everling.   PAGE 85 (BOTTOM): J. E. Goldthwaite et al., *Body Mechanics in the Study and Treatment of Disease*, Lippincott, 1934. PAGE 88: F. Everling.   PAGE 89 (TOP): Heka Davis.   PAGE 92: Photograph by Frances Flaherty, courtesy Flaherty Study Center.   PAGE 102 (BOTTOM, RIGHT): Paul B. Herbert.   PAGE 105: Ylla, Lausanne, 1954. Rapho Guillumette Pictures.   PAGE 135: Alissa Goldring.   PAGE 157: Paul B. Herbert.   PAGES 163, 164: Teri Modlin.   PAGE 172 (TOP), Photo Mariann Reismann, from Dr. Emmi Pikler, *Que sait faire votre bébé*, Les Editeurs Français Réunis, 1951.   PAGE 177: M. A. Roche.   PAGE 204: B. Moosbrugger. Rietberg Museum, Zurich.   PAGE 215: "Hollyhock," by Arthur Dove.   PAGE 230: Sophie Ludwig.

I have no parents:
I make the heavens and earth my parents.
I have no home:
I make awareness my home.
I have no life or death:
I make the tides of breathing my life and death.
I have no divine power:
I make honesty my divine power.
I have no means:
I make understanding my means.
I have no magic secrets:
I make character my magic secret.
I have no body:
I make endurance my body.
I have no eyes:
I make the flash of lightning my eyes.
I have no ears:
I make sensibility my ears.
I have no limbs:
I make promptness my limbs.
I have no strategy:
I make "unshadowed by thought" my strategy.
I have no designs:
I make "seizing opportunity by the forelock" my design.
I have no miracles:
I make right-action my miracles.
I have no principles:
I make adaptability to all circumstances my principles.
I have no tactics:
I make emptiness and fullness my tactics.
I have no talents:
I make ready wit my talent.
I have no friends:
I make my mind my friend.
I have no enemy:
I make carelessness my enemy.
I have no armor:
I make benevolence and righteousness my armor.
I have no castle:
I make immovable-mind my castle.
I have no sword:
I make absence of self my sword.

—Anonymous samurai, 14th century

Contents

Toward a More Sensitive Relating / 91

Epilogue / 223

Appendices / 227

AUTHOR'S NOTE

In some three years of intermittent work, I have finally written a book that attempts to convey the nonverbal substance of the exceedingly subtle and deep work to which my wife, Charlotte Selver, has devoted her life. I have revised it many times, aided by suggestions she has made. In the process of these revisions, we have found that the experience of sensory awareness is so individual that any attempt to bring it into words must necessarily reveal the one who makes the attempt in his own unique character and approach to living. There are therefore many instances in which I have not followed Charlotte's advice but have made bold to assert my own views and my experience, with all the intellectual and literary background which I carry with me—a background with which I must constantly struggle in such an undertaking.

Nevertheless, I feel there is much here that will be recognized as real and down to earth. The great bulk of this comes from Charlotte. With negligible exceptions, the experiments described are her experiments, the questions her questions. If here and there I have had the good fortune to evoke some of the living context in which these experiments and questions come alive, it is through the reliving of her classes, which have been the major force in my life for the last fifteen years.

This is part autobiography, part philosophy, part guidebook for the student of sensory awareness, and part a fair equivalent in words of actual experience. Taken altogether, it is my sense of this work, as fully and clearly as I can state it now.

I never knew the teacher whom Charlotte revered and to whom she feels she owes her entire work. I know only Charlotte,

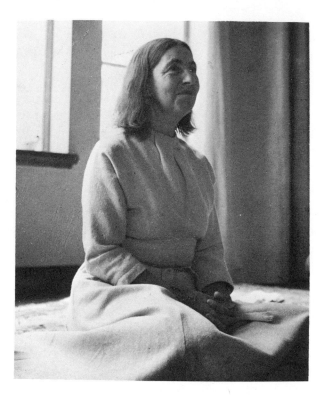

and to me this work is hers. Perhaps someday it will be the work of many people—it is already that of an increasing number—for it is a work of love and of reality.

I am much indebted to a number of friends for helpful suggestions: Richard Baker-roshi, of the San Francisco Zen Center; Professor Allen Walker Read and Charlotte Read; Dr. Bernard Weitzman; Connie Siegel; Dr. Edward Deci; Dr. Jorge Derbez; my editor, Stuart Miller. I am very grateful to the late Alan Watts for his encouragement.

Above all, I must thank Bill Littlewood for tempering the alloy from which this instrument was forged. Without the love, the clarity, and the endurance that guided his often Spartan hand, it would have rung far less true than it does now.

Monhegan, Maine, 1973

Introduction

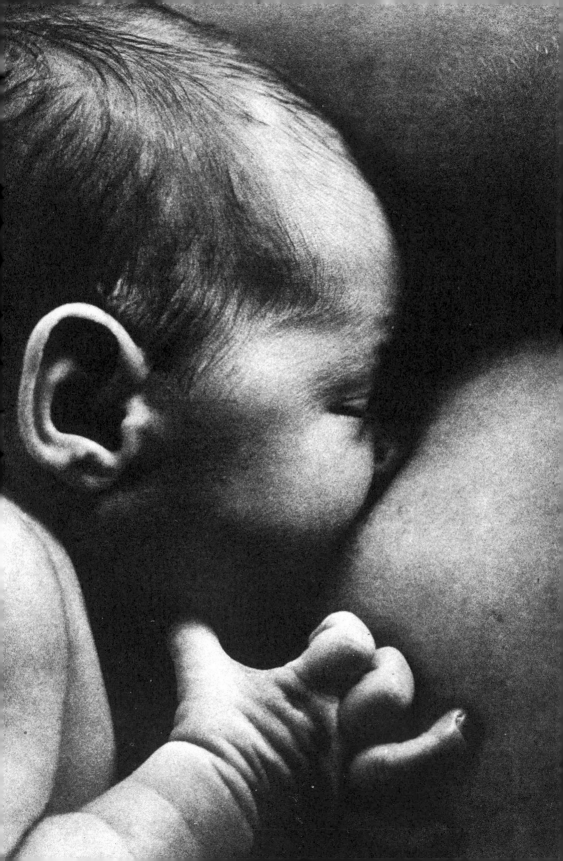

1 BEING IN THE WORLD

After heavy rains last week, we planted seeds in our garden. They are sprouting already. I know from past exploration how deep and intimately the little roots are pushing their way, with the amazing vigor of infancy, down through the dense particles of soil; and as I look I can almost see the stems and leaflets unfolding in the same air that I feel bathing me inside and out, under the same sun that beats on my skin. It sets me to considering the subject of this book.

Does not all individual life, as with these seeds, begin in moisture—either in the sea or, as here, in the damp earth, or on the yolk of an egg, or in the fluids of the womb? In the womb, when the united cells multiply to the point where something that one could call consciousness infuses them, the whole development of the new organism continues to take place in that total, invisible immediacy of the environment which is the nature of fluid, which leaves no crack unentered, no surface unembraced.

Until birth we had no experience of distance: of the possibility of falling, of the sound of something not adjacent to us, of warmth either coming to us or going from us. No wonder that on entering the world outside we clutched at the breast, with its soft tissues like our own, and breathed the strange air more easily when held and enveloped in mother's arms.

In this new world, it was for the first time possible—indeed, necessary—to be alone: mother might be here or absent. Gradually, new-found doors began opening. Sounds came and went, which little by little could be related to phenomena outside ourselves; smells likewise; what we touched, and what

touched us, was always changing. Finally the growing kaleido-
scope before our eyes began separating into enduring, recog-
nizable forms, nearer or farther, with each of which we could
have a different connection.

Though the nerve ends in our skin were in immediate contact only with the air, or with the delicious water of our bath,
or here and there with clothing, crib, and playthings, or now
and then with mother, still we were not out of touch with the
world in the distance. We could hear mother's voice from afar
and see her when we could not touch her, and we smiled in
recognition and pleasure. Indeed, we had a voice too, which
could go out to others and arouse perceptible reactions in them;
and we had hands and feet with which we could reach out to
grasp or kick objects in space. As our enlarging consciousness
embraced a larger and more differentiated world, both near
and far, in the embrace itself was contact, though of varying
kinds. The shape or color which we could not reach was yet in
our eye, the voice was in our ear, the smell in our nostrils.

Gradually, new-found doors began opening.

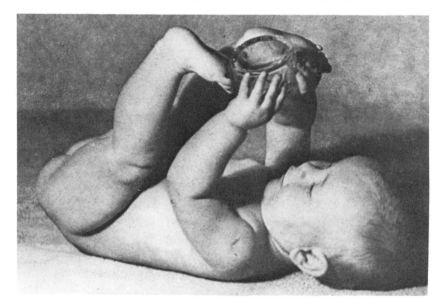

And now came a new contact and immediacy as we gained experience and began storing the past to give larger meaning to the present. When we saw and smelled mother and heard her voice, memory was there, and our stomach began to contract in hunger for her milk and our skin to yearn for her touch. And the future entered. When we were already hungry, as mother appeared, the comfort which had not yet reached us brought our smile of anticipation, as a kitten purrs before the milk is poured.

Time and space, which had no existence in the womb, appear gradually to the growing child and to the adult as being everywhere and part of everything, so as to define all objects of perception. Yet they bring with them no necessity of separateness, except in the particular. This or that phenomenon is now with us and now apart from us, but the stream of phenomena still envelops us as did the fluids of the womb. There is no natural necessity that keeps us from living our lives as immediately and fully in touch with our environment as any fish in water, or any deer in the woods, or any plant in our garden.

But all the while that we were developing our connection with the world, something else was forming in us quite without parallel in any other living creatures. What had been a few cells, then a few thousand, then a few million, were proliferating by the billions in our brain to receive the messages, relate and organize them, regulate reactions to them; and the head which housed these cells was so heavy and unwieldy that, for us alone among creatures, its movement and rest were a primary concern throughout our infancy.

It is our fate that it must be a primary concern to us throughout our lives. For in the superlatively developed cortex of our brains lies another seed[1]—that of most of our human *doing*,[2]

1. Cf. A. T. W. Simeons, *Man's Presumptuous Brain* (New York: Dutton, 1961). Also L. L. Whyte, *The Next Development in Man* (New York: Holt, 1948).
2. Since writing these lines, I have read Carlos Castaneda's *A Separate Reality* and *Journey to Ixtlan* (New York: Simon and Schuster, 1971 and 1972) no fewer than five times each. His talk of *doing* and *not-doing* does not refer to purposeful activities, as does my reference here, but to an entirely unconscious interpretation of perceptions in conventional terms. These processes seem to me, however, to be so

and of our undoing. Our unique human faculty of developing animal vocalizations into the fixed symbols of words and our fleeting perceptions into circumscribed concepts has given us a second plane of reality, the conventional, which because of its endless conveniences comes to supplant, or at least ·to veil, the original. For the original can never be captured and possessed, but only indicated.

The abstract thought and language from which all our concepts arise have made the civilized world possible. They have divided experience into fragments, of which so many can be clearly identified, agreed upon, and used that from the perceptions of a myriad of individuals could be compiled the encyclopedia, and from the selected elements of the earth could be constructed New York City. This seems to be possible only for human beings. Animals, relying directly on their senses, can often communicate perceptions and feelings as well as we. Like us, they doubtless divide the world, in practical ways, into the secure and the dangerous, the useful and useless. But lacking the brain that might evolve a language to freeze these divisions into abstractions, they cannot build consciously, as we do, on the past, or share our social achievements. They can only relate directly to the ever-changing present—either fully and healthily, or sometimes, if so conditioned by us, neurotically. By the same token, in their wild state at least, they are spared the alienation from nature and the loss of integrity which beset mankind—encyclopedia, New York, and all— divided between what we perceive and what we think about it.

Like Hamlet's, our world has become sicklied with thought. We do not refer to our own experience but to our overwhelming legacy of the conceptualizations of others. Instead of occupying our infinite talents in procuring our few simple needs, or in molding and weaving the earth as do the lilies of the field, we are endlessly correcting and tampering with the world, and perhaps, in our explosive exploitation, only making it worse. How can we do otherwise? For if our actions derive ultimately

---

closely related, and Castaneda's understanding of them to be so direct and profound, that for this, as for many other reasons, I would put his books at the very head of my personal bibliography.

from our beliefs—i.e., our *concepts*—we are forever manipulating a world which we do not directly perceive and therefore cannot know.

During my life, I have often rejected one authority only to accept another. Underneath, I was afraid at the thought of living in a world where there was not Someone, somewhat like myself, who *knew*. But I have now come to feel that, to know what one is doing with life, it is no use to consult authorities. It is precisely through the veils which authorities have spun for us that our own ears and eyes and nerves must begin to penetrate if our hands are to grasp the world and our hearts to feel it. We must recover our own capacity to taste for ourselves. Then we shall be able to judge also.

This calls for discipline. One discipline to control the rampant mind has been evolved in Zen[3] and other forms of Buddhist meditation. Another, if I dare speak of it in such august company, is the subject of this book.

---

3. See Appendix B.

2 COMING TO OUR SENSES

The work which I shall be presenting here—the life work, first, of Elsa Gindler and then, as it has come to me and to many hundreds of others, of Charlotte Selver[1]—has been spread in the last decade throughout growth centers in the United States under the heading "Work on the Body." Yet when Charlotte and I were invited recently to contribute a chapter on this work, it was to a symposium entitled *Workshops of the Mind*.[2]

This contradiction brings up a special difficulty, as persistent as it is annoying, to which I should like to devote a few words at the very beginning of things.

The venerable division of the person into the psychic and the somatic seems to me to be strongly challenged by such an expression as "sensory awareness," in which the prime psychic characteristic of awareness is proposed in somatic terms. This is possible, I believe, because the division is of purely cultural origin, without biological validity.

I know very well that this division as generally conceived today—the so-called "mind-body split"—refers to the immense and still-growing separation in our culture between intellectual processes and sensory experience. No one can doubt that this is a catastrophic fact. On one hand, we have the abstract information, as well as the theories, clichés, stereotypes, and fantasies, that are the stock in trade of most people's conversation, reading, writing, and trains of thought—in a word, of their consciousness. On the other hand is experience, which for a

1. See Appendix A for notes on Elsa Gindler and Heinrich Jacoby and for Charlotte Selver's introduction of this work into the United States.
2. Bernard Aaronson, *Workshops of the Mind* (New York: Doubleday, 1975).

great many people today is practically limited to comfort and discomfort.

But how "mind" has come to be identified with the intellectual and "body" with the experiential is a question that might inspire a fascinating history of thought and culture. In such a division of things, the whole world of art, music, poetry, meditation, and love would have no place.

As a stop-gap, I am going to suggest a semantic relief for this difficulty: namely, that the terms "body" and "mind" might represent quite different categories of thought which could not properly be put into opposition. I have not always thought so. I, too, grew up speaking of "bodily functions" as referring, for instance, to perspiration or bowel movement, but never to reason or understanding, and classing as "mental functions" arithmetic or spelling, but never hockey or dance. Now, still staying with the English language, I think of my "body" as of a dimension, in the same sense in which one speaks of a body of water. There is certainly a vital difference between my body and a body of water, but it lies in the fact that my body lays out the boundaries of an *organism*—or organization of interdependent tissues, none of which can be separated from the others without the loss of its whole reason for existence. This organism, visibly and in other perceptual ways definable as a body, has functions: e.g., metabolism, respiration, circulation, et cetera, and *mind*. Mind, in this light, could no more be contrasted to body than metabolism could. When either the mind, which correlates our reactions, or the metabolism, which produces our temperature, begins to cease functioning, that is the end of us—except to the extent that we can be kept "alive" like tissue in a test tube.

But there is another, far more emotionally charged, significance to this division: the long human history of dividing the person into body and soul. "The hopes and fears of all the years" are related to this—the ancient opposition between the "lusts of the flesh" and the "aspirations of the spirit." But the origins of both the words "aspiration" and "spirit" refer to breathing; and is it not the flesh that breathes?

Are we then to understand this division of the person into

mind and body as a practical human artifice, or as a description of reality, in which "mind" or "spirit" might control or yield to the "body," or in which the "soul," in death or otherwise, might maintain its own separate existence?

Why do we not divide animals so? Their brains are smaller, but their hearts can be as loving and their eyes as "soulful" as ours.[3] With no abstract good and evil, animals take what comes and suffer without resentment. Though filled with fears of real dangers, they have no fear of death. Living to the full, they have no need of a future—a fact we instinctively realize when we tell our child, mourning his dead pet and asking if it will go to heaven, that, however intelligent animals may be, they have no souls and do not go to heaven.

■   A conception of consciousness as simply a function of any organization of living cells, ranging in complexity from the reactivity of an amoeba to the genius of a Goethe or a Beethoven, leaves us free to disregard such puzzling and troublesome questions as being of conventional and semantic origin and not concerning the real matter of living. Any work in awareness grounded in such an understanding necessarily directs itself to the whole person, rather than to any fraction of him. To separate and seek out the "spiritual" or the "physical" is no longer relevant.[4]

But are not we in this work precisely separating and seeking out that awareness we qualify as *sensory*, and thereby diminishing ourselves? I say no. There is no other direct awareness, even though our so-called "five senses" are also just conceptual abstractions from the totality of our sentience. We are seeking the sensory foundation for what may be our many intellectual edifices, our connection and relationship to the enduring, if ever-changing, earth; for only on such a foundation can any organic superstructure arise.

3. CF. note page 109.
4. This conception of consciousness is my understanding of Teilhard de Chardin's *The Phenomenon of Man* (New York: Harper, 1969). Whether or not I have understood him aright, and whatever similar or different conclusions it may lead us to, this is the first time my own intuitions in this matter have been satisfactorily formulated.

There is no lack of information in America, but one may say that there is too little personal knowledge of anything except isolated facts and mechanical and social processes. Our emphasis on the sensory will not diminish us. It will refine and enlarge us.

■   What might be the awareness of one of the seedlings growing in our garden, perceiving and reacting to light and darkness, moisture and drought, warmth and cold —its roots ceaselessly exploring downward, while stem and leaves explore upward, everything seeking to satisfy its needs, the whole constantly tending outward, until finally one day it will unfold in blossoms and dry up in seeds? The image of blossoming captivates us, and we speak of knowing others by their fruits. Have we, too, an organic nature, striving plant-like to explore in all directions, and bursting from the confining structure of concepts and images we have inherited? Our grandfathers often felt they had spirits striving to free themselves of fleshly bonds. Are we not flesh, perhaps, striving to free ourselves of intellectual bonds? For if we consider flesh neurologically, chemically, functionally, it surely represents the most "spiritual" aspect of the cosmos!

One may say that, like plants, we are sentient; like animals, we are sentient and intelligent. Unlike these, we are also intellectual. That is why one might accept the term "sensory awareness" as most closely indicating the relationship which we share with other living beings and which, as I shall attempt to show, is by no means less than human.

■   Our study of sensing is simply a study of consciousness. One can come to feel when consciousness is occupied with thoughts, and when these thoughts arise organically from our perceptions, or are disconnected and distracting trains of association. We can tell when we are open to the reality of the moment and when, in anxiety or in our efforts at control, we close ourselves. We can sense when consciousness flows freely, and when it meets obstacles and stops or wavers.

In our study, we come to realize that it is through consciousness that we can allow a meaningful connection with what we

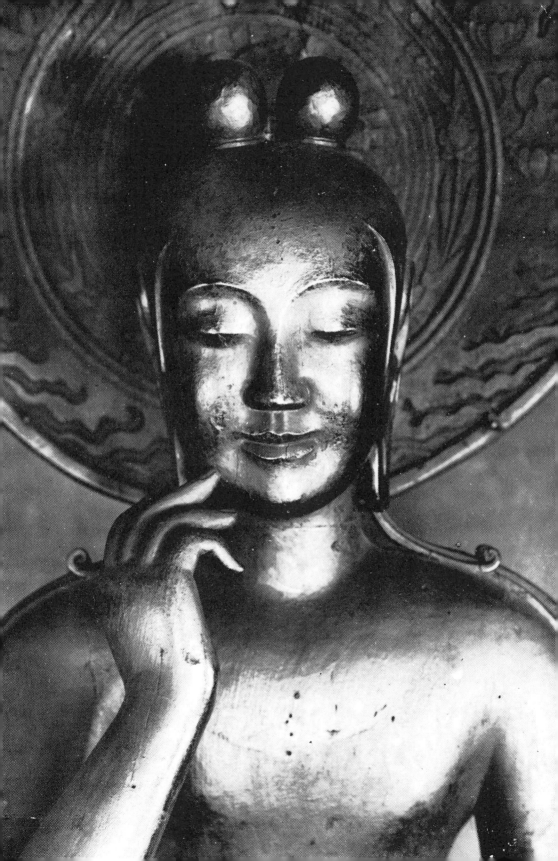

approach and what we do, as distinguished from the "blind" or "insensate" or mechanical ways in which we so often interact with our environment. We recognize that clarity of perception underlies all understanding and all intelligent behavior. The saying "Buddha is in everyone" can be understood as referring not to any separate divinity, but to the potential of full consciousness in every organism according to its nature. This would restore to the organs of consciousness, our senses, the dignity which is due them. It would permit us to live securely in our real perceptions, shallow or deep as the case might be, but free of our never-ending speculations.

"Buddha is in everyone."

3 NATURE AND "SECOND NATURE"

Like Zen meditation,[1] sensory awareness is not a teaching but a *practice*.
Though we act on Elsa Gindler's recognition that there is a
natural tendency to order in the functioning and growth of the
human organism,[2] we have no real theoretical framework, and
our experiments are entirely empirical. Our aim is not the
acquisition of skills, but the freedom to explore sensitively and
to learn from exploration. We propose experiments and ask
questions directed toward the possibility of *experiencing*.

In the classes, new recognitions and new attitudes come
about as a result of the student's own explorations, which he
must go into for himself, at his own pace, even though working
as a member of a group. We neither instruct verbally nor offer
an example to imitate. We merely work with practical means
toward an adult version of the quiet, open, curious attitude
which healthy children have to the world they are born into—a
world they never tire of investigating. The child does not separate himself from his world but is just as curious about his own
processes as about any others. Similarly, the attitude we seek is
neither extraverted nor introverted, but one of openness and
consciousness generally. We try to allow whatever becomes
conscious in our present state the time it needs to become
clearer to us.

In this work, we come gradually to distinguish perception
from such other elements of consciousness as thought, fantasy,
image, and emotion, each of which may push to occupy the
stage. These normal human functions have in many of us

1. See Appendix B.   2. See Appendix A.

become separated from the experience to which they belong and now hover in us ready to attach themselves to whatever appears; so that the state of mind of many people today is something like an orchestra in which each member would be playing from a different score. In the current therapies of the Humanistic movement, there is much concern with extricating these different functions from the tangle they are in. Work is done on the release of blocked emotions, on the freeing and accepting of fantasy, on the self-image, et cetera. Our work, not intended to be therapeutic, has none of these objectives. Nevertheless, as we come to more inner quiet and clarity, a great deal happens by itself which in this light might be considered therapeutic.

The advance toward clearer perception and more authentic experience does not lack emotion, any more than the note

---

**Just as curious about his own processes
as about any others.**

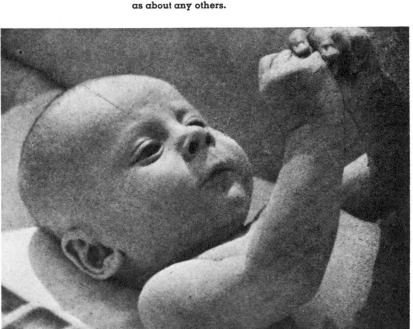

struck clearly on a violin lacks overtones. Nor need the clarity
of a sensation suffer when it blossoms into thought or form.
When it is spoken out, it may be poetry; when set down on
canvas, it may be pure expression. But to *seek* for sensation is
to seek for the pot of gold at the foot of the rainbow, and the
emotional release that is *sought for* is elusive and obscure.

And what we very often mean by "thinking"—the repeti-
tive, compulsive occupation of consciousness with loose associations, clichés, and calculations—leads us, not toward, but away
from fuller consciousness. This kind of "thinking" is indeed the
anesthetic and narcotic drug to which so much in our established culture is constantly leading us, and to which we have
become addicted since childhood. Withdrawal from it, if not as
painful as from heroin, is surely as difficult, as every person
seeking peace of mind must have discovered. Yet paradoxically,
as the young people have found, to the consternation of their
elders, it is the virtue of the so-called psychedelic drugs that
with their help this narcotic thinking can often be laid to rest.
Then, as in the Zen saying, the waters can become still and the
moon be reflected clearly. We seek this stillness too, though on
a disciplined and organismic basis rather than a pharmaceuti-
cal one.

Attention to sensing quiets what is compulsive in our
thought, so that the mind becomes free and available for its
normal function of perception. When the radio in the mind is
stilled, everything else can come to life. The camper's lantern
is blown out, and the darkness fills with stars as the woods
deepen and widen for him. The primitive world in which things
appear and disappear, bloom and fade, eat and are eaten can be
perceived surrounding us—and including us. I myself have
feared this world, in which I have had little practice in living. I
have spent much of my life in the half make-believe world of
words and know that, though it may often bore one, it is comfortable, and one is loath to give it up. This is the familiar and
the "secure," even in its insecurity. When it seems inadequate,
one can always dwell in the past or add a new dimension like
heaven, or tomorrow. In the world of perception the present is
infinite; the only authority is I, the perceiver. We cannot know

the future, and only the least trace of the past. But when we breathe the air of the night woods, and let their forms and almost imperceptible sounds into us, or when we stand silent in the sunlight that glows on rocks and leaves and city buildings, and perhaps feel the earth sustaining us, we know that we exist, at first hand, surrounded by innumerable other beings who exist too. Need we ask more?

The study of this work is our whole organismic functioning in the world we perceive, of which we are a part—our personal ecology: how we go about our activities, how we relate to people, to situations, to objects. We aim to discover what is natural in this functioning and what is conditioned: what is our nature, which evolution has designed to keep us in touch with the rest of the world, and what has become our "second nature," as Charlotte likes to call it, which tends to keep us apart. We shall discover a spectrum spreading from the perceived to the conceived, in which our upbringing has found us at one end and pushed us to the other, where it has held us. In sensing, we shall gradually return to that broad area in the center of the spectrum where our birthright is balanced with our culture, and from where we are freer to move in any direction.

4 THE FINGER POINTING TO THE MOON

I believe it can fairly be said of work in sensory awareness that the longer a person has been leading groups, the less easy it is to catalogue what he does. Charlotte, who has been working more than forty years, is constantly improvising and coming on approaches that she has not tried before. For the things we do become less and less *techniques* as one matures, and serve more and more as improvisations in which each participant in a class simply gains practice in coming to his own experience.

It will therefore be important to remember that the following descriptions in no sense constitute a manual and will only lead into blind alleys if followed mechanically. Of course, this has already happened, over and over. Young teachers, seeking more eclectic and comprehensive approaches, have "integrated" sensory-awareness "techniques" into their methods. But there are no more techniques in this study than there are in love. One cannot "integrate" fresh air into a stuffy room. One lets the fresh air in, and in its own time the staleness leaves. Whoever immerses himself in this study will change, without any effort or intention to do so, and the change will express itself in all his activities.

In this light, it will be understood when I say that classes seldom take place and follow sequences quite as I shall present them. This book is a distillation and a blending. To present our work *verbatim* is a task for the future—though, indeed, I hope for the very near future[1]—an unearthing from the hundreds of hours of existing tapes. If this account seems to offer a blue-

1. Beginnings have already been made by Benjamin Weaver and by the Charlotte Selver Foundation. Cf. Appendix A.

print, it will have failed. Its intention is merely to convey an attitude.

Over the years, Charlotte Selver has chosen numerous titles for her courses and seminars. There are no self-evident titles, as in a school curriculum. As with an abstract painting, or with music or dance, a title, when it is not just an identification for practical convenience, is a cue to the uninterpretable. It is a verbalization of precisely that which in its nature is non-verbal. In that beautiful Japanese image, it is a finger pointing to the moon.

One might say something similar of this entire book.

The title of one of Charlotte's early courses in the New School for Social Research, in New York, was "Walking, Standing, Sitting, Lying: The Four Dignities of Man." I have taken this ancient Chinese saying as a heading for the first part of my description of the work, even though my treatment of this fourfold subject reflects the practical limitations of working conditions, as a glance at the table of contents will reveal.

Other titles have been "Study of Breathing"; "Being All There"; "Nonverbal Experience and Communication"; "Awake, Tune In: Unfold"; "Toward Expanded Consciousness"; "Meditation in Everyday Living"; "Contact versus Technique and Manipulation"; "Giving and Receiving"; "Entering Experience in Depth"; "Opening Doors"; "Toward a More Sensitive Relating"; "The Delight of Immediacy."

It might be useful if one glanced now and then at these titles while reading the descriptions below, for with few exceptions every class is concerned with all of them. They are not titles of different courses, but different aspects of a single study. There is the further consideration, as I have already hinted, that we are not seeking a *correct* standing, sitting, breathing, et cetera, according to any pre-established criterion, but are simply studying the nature of the phenomenon itself as it occurs in each of us individually. What is it that is really happening when we say we are "standing" or "breathing"? Since we do not seek a verbal or in any way definitive answer, this is a study without certifiable achievement and without end. Its only interest is the essential interest in living processes themselves. In it the humblest student, though he may lack clarity and depth, has as much authority as the most experienced teacher.

With these cautions, I shall now try to give a taste of some of the basic and representative activities which we are constantly exploring.

The Four Dignities of Man

5 THE SEARCH FOR STANDING

Our workshops normally take place in a large, bare room with mats or carpeting. The quieter and friendlier the better. Shoes, handbags, and the like are left outside, and participants are dressed comfortably for sitting on the floor (our home base) and for unhampered movement.

Charlotte's way of beginning is unpredictable; mine less so. After a few explanations, I usually just ask the group to "come to standing."

This is an invitation to one of the commonest activities of daily living, which perhaps more than any other distinguishes man from animals, but which our culture does not recognize as an activity at all. To the participants, it simply means to stand up—something they have done many thousands of times, indeed something they have been *told* to do a thousand times, often with rewards and penalties attached. In actuality, what usually occurs is that one either jumps up; dutifully, perhaps resentfully, pushes or drags oneself up; struggles to rise; or rises as one has learned in calisthenics or dance, with some special technique—all of which has become second nature and more or less unconscious. Whatever happens, it seldom fails to involve visible effort. It is a practical certainty that hardly anyone, since infancy, has consciously and sensitively *come to standing*.

Who, in adulthood, comes to standing consciously, for its own sake, unless for the relief of "stretching one's legs"? Indeed who, unless sick or injured, takes the trouble to feel his way to standing at all?

Yet when a house has been brought to standing, a rooftree

is raised and there is general celebration, just as on that great occasion in the family when for the first time the child, who has lain and sat and crawled, finally is seen standing freely on the ground, with no other support. At least this is the case when houses, and children, have real significance. We shall work on this question for months and years, for we must endlessly rediscover in ourselves the difference between the constructed building, which we aim to have erected in the most trustworthy method and with the most approved techniques, and the living

For the first time the child is seen standing freely on the ground, with no other support.

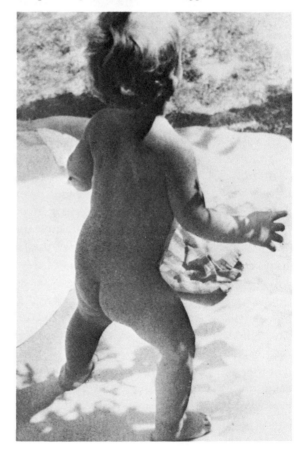

creature, who must find his way each time anew. When this distinction becomes real to us, we can never tire of exploring it.

We have asked people to enter the work without expectations, but this is asking a good deal. Probably they will stand more or less patiently waiting for something to happen. Few in the group are conscious that a great deal is already going on inside them, for they are waiting for a cue from the outside.

What will happen if we request the group to shut off the main avenue to the outside and stand with eyes closed?

This is quite a step. Immediately there are reactions. A number of people will feel a loss of balance and the need for something to hold on to, which is remedied when they allow a peep again. It becomes clear that these people have been relying on their eyes for *support*.

For most of us, indeed, the visual has been much over-emphasized. We have been exhorted to "see," "look," and "watch" since infancy, but seldom to *feel out* a situation. Closing the eyes may bring restfulness to some, but to others it will bring insecurity; still others, who have no difficulty standing, may nevertheless experience a vague anxiety. Since childhood, we have also been warned to "look out!" For many of us a new element has introduced itself, though perhaps unconsciously: *is it safe?*

So much about our whole way of living may be called into question by this simple experiment that a few people may be unable to close their eyes at all.[1] For others, standing may become quite uncomfortable, especially if they continue to stand out of vanity or obedience. But if we can stay with it for a while, something may be discovered. For one thing, if the question is raised, we may quite possibly find that closing the eyes has by no means ended the attempt to see, and that behind closed lids the eyes have remained very active.

If asked whether our eyelids are *resting* over our eyes, or whether efforts are needed to keep them closed, we will very often discover that we are actually struggling to look through eyelids dutifully held closed.

1. There are cases where this inability has survived literally years of work.

At this point, one may either open the eyes to find relief, or, recognizing the contradiction in one's activities, give up something of the urge to see, which immediately reduces the efforts in eyes and eyelids and makes one feel easier altogether. In the latter case, there may be the interesting discovery that, simply in becoming conscious, a previously unconscious inner conflict may dissolve, freeing energies for coming to more balance and fuller standing. The recognition may come to one: *I don't have to use my eyes for standing; I can sense.*

An entirely new feeling of security and potency may come from such recognitions, and a delicious sense of one's own being, even at the very beginning of our study. It may be felt that even in such minute muscles as those around the eyes energies can be bound which halt whole processes in the organism, restrict breathing, and preoccupy consciousness. Even purely rational processes may be involved, as in the

---

I don't have to use my eyes for standing; I can sense.

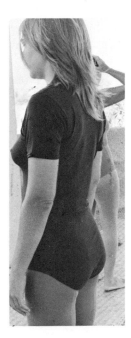

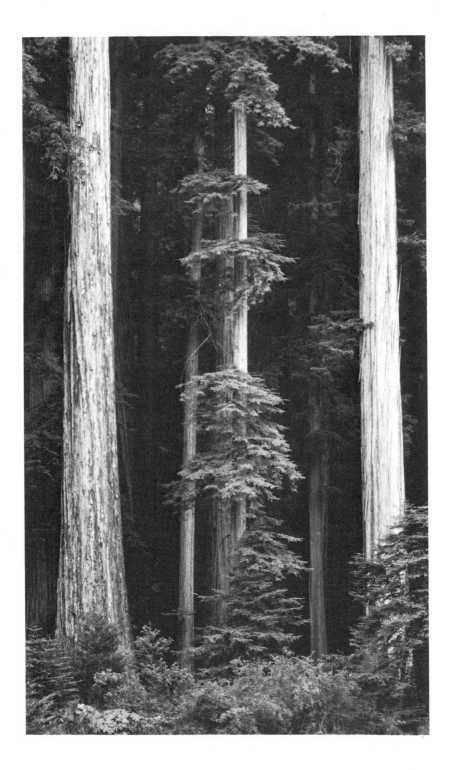

realization that in closing one's eyes in the first place, the perhaps unconscious decision was justified that no danger was present. This is not "body work," as it is so often called, but an awakening of the person. And when we finally open our eyes and perhaps find that, at least for the moment, we can *continue* to stand, simply seeing, without using our eyes for help, the sense of being may increase still further.

In the first moments of work, by inquiring into the function of seeing in simple standing, we have plunged into one of the most difficult and persistent human conditionings. But another question, equally important and perhaps closely related, is apt to be raised when some student remarks that he feels .his watching eyes have something to do with thinking. Very likely, others in the class will agree; several may report that they found themselves as distracted by their thoughts as by their watchfulness.

Now it is no use, when a person's eyes are closed, to tell him to stop looking. That just invites a new inner attempt at control, which is what the looking is in the first place. One can raise the question; and when he is able, he will find it very relieving to give it up. It is equally useless to tell him to stop thinking. But one may ask if the person can feel himself thinking, and how it would feel to permit more resting in his mind. Does anything new come to consciousness if thoughts come more to quiet?

We may also ask: is one fixing one's attention on difficulties and attempting to correct them? And if so, how would it be simply to stay uncritical and open for whatever inner changes might happen by themselves?

I need hardly say what a change in our usual attitude this would involve. Our whole education has been concerned with analyzing difficulties, remembering other people's admonitions, and making corrections. Now it is suggested that merely by allowing more consciousness we might be giving things the possibility of resolving themselves. Besides this, there is the special problem with standing that we have been told often enough that it is "just standing," and is boring and fatiguing— which, when we have heard it from people we esteem, actually tends to make it so. Would it not be somehow disloyal of us to find it otherwise?

For many reasons, then, these few minutes of standing may have become quite tiring for certain people, while for others discoveries may have been made that require time to digest. This is the time for lying down and resting for a while. Afterward, those who have made discoveries may enjoy sharing them, while those who have felt "nothing" will be relieved by saying so.

6 STANDING AS RELATING

Thus far, all of our attention has been turned inward. But if we continue a little longer with work on standing, a new direction may be opened, drawing the attention away from the inner and toward the outer. The leader may ask, "Do you feel what you are standing on?"—thus appealing directly to the sensory nerves in the feet.

Since we have left our shoes outside and many will be barefoot, this is an invitation to sensing which, for a surprising number of people, has not really been practiced since childhood. The feet are by nature very sensitive—even sensual—and many people will respond with interest. They do feel the floor and its coverings. They begin to discover textures, temperatures, the solidity under them. Something is really there which they had taken for granted but had not experienced.

After a while, we may ask, "If you feel the floor, how are you relating to it?"

Now who has asked such a question of himself? Does one relate to a floor? We allow time for the question to sink in.

It may help to be more specific. "Are you simply standing on the floor—with your whole foot?"

Again people begin to make discoveries. When they report later what they found, it will turn out that some were standing mainly on their heels—perhaps as though holding back from something—and felt themselves not simply standing but also *pressing*. When they allowed a more fully distributed standing, in which more of the foot could participate, there were sometimes unfamiliar and exciting sensations of fuller presence and connection. Others found the opposite: they were as though poised on the balls of their feet, eager to go forward; and in this they were pressing on the floor and not just standing either. The report of one stimulates recollections in the others. Someone found he was trying to grip the floor with his toes, another that his toes had been avoiding the floor. We may emphasize the discovery, but we refrain from any suggestion or interpretation. That is the student's business, not ours. Yet now and then someone glimpses that he has a tendency to hold back or push forward in many situations. When he realizes this, it is because he is ripe for it, not because we have tampered with him; and it can have the force of genuine recognition.

The feet begin to discover textures, temperatures.

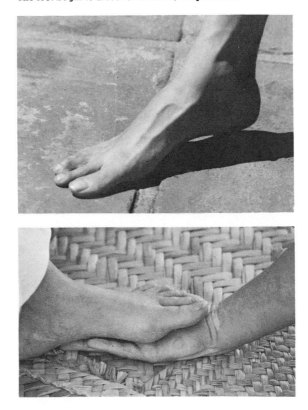

If standing is a task that calls for clear perception of the support under one, and a clearly functional response to this support, could one speak of the foot as reacting not only sensitively but even intelligently? Can one *identify* one's foot with oneself? Is "foot" indeed just an abstraction of speech, so that we are not really sensing and reacting through our feet, as we might through such actual possessions as skis or stilts, but rather simply functioning consciously all the way down to where we reach the ground?

Do we *stand on our own feet*, as we have so often been exhorted to, or do we stand *on the floor*?

Very much may begin to become conscious to those who can live with such favorite questions of Charlotte's, which can never be answered except as regards the present moment, and even then seldom with a categorical yes or no—questions which may be asked at the very outset, and which may well continue to be asked to the end of one's life.

7 A FEW DIFFICULTIES

If our questions have caught a beginner's interest, the workshop has been launched. Clearly the genuineness of the questions, as well as their sequence and timing, is important. If they are just chosen from notes we have preassembled, they may seem artificial to the participant, unless, as often happens, he has come so persuaded of the esoteric value of the work, or of the leader, that he will accept anything.

But if the questions arise from what the leader perceives of the actual situation, they will be felt by the others and may then have a compelling authenticity. The participant may realize that for once he is being asked something that he alone can answer—not something that depends on information or definition. The question is not, is it a flat earth or a round, spinning earth that is beneath me; not even, is it carpet, or wood, or concrete; but is there *something* beneath me? Not what I have heard about it, but *what I feel*. For instance, will it support me—i.e., *does* it support me? Is it cold or warm, hard or soft? Does it accept me? Do I accept it?

The realization that the answers to such questions may be constantly changing—that what felt hard and cold may become warm and soft, or vice versa—makes them none the less authentic. On the contrary, it may lead to the insight that perception is relative, an insight generally repugnant to our institutions, and have far-reaching consequences. In such cases, occurring not infrequently, one experiences the unfolding of sensory awareness into the beginning of wisdom.

Of course, it all goes much more slowly than I make it seem. An honest question may merely set up a conflict in the hearer's mind, for he has been conditioned to be conscious of what he has been taught, not of what his senses bring to him. An example of this is the participant's unfailing tendency to translate the leader's questions into terms familiar to him. For instance, "Do you allow your eyes to rest?" becomes "Think of your eyes." "Do you let the floor support you?" becomes "Let the floor support you." He has learned since childhood to belittle his own experience and "learn from the experience of others"—i.e., to supplant his experience with intellectual processes pleasing to the teacher. If he is now to dare to experience strongly enough so that this pattern of repression and transformation may begin to dissolve, we must go slowly and quietly. He must have plenty of time and be free from any eagerness on the part of the leader. Otherwise, barriers to experience may be broken through without being perceived or understood and, like ice on puddles, will re-form overnight.

Beginners may in any case feel a little hesitant to speak out. Perhaps someone remembers that he suddenly found himself holding his breath: is such a trifle something to report? Or that the floor became less hard: might that not sound absurd? Or that he felt a stiffness in his back, or in his mind's eye saw an image of himself standing: could this be interesting to anyone? Besides, people are always talking, and this was supposed to be a nonverbal workshop.

But when the first person gets the courage to speak out, he finds that others listen. Details of real experience are interesting, no matter how "trifling." The others begin to speak too. It becomes apparent that the group, in its halting, unpracticed way, has actually been exploring a situation. Someone may now announce that he has found himself "one with the all," or has left his body and been floating weightlessly. We are confronted with the sirens of *idea* and *image*, for whom plain sensation is not enough and who will turn up to entice us from our way the whole length of the voyage.

With a mature leader, each workshop and each session will be unique. Each beginning has its own inner dynamic, its own set of genes, which the leader may or may not sense. When the leader, sensing this dynamic, is not ambitious, but is able to permit it to unfold, rather than follow the familiar course of control and manipulation, the session will have life and validity. For he is not a leader, when he is working well, but rather a guide, exploring and discovering with the others obscure regions with which he is perhaps only somewhat more familiar than they. To the extent that he takes over, even in the direction of his own image of spontaneity, the validity is diminished. The most precious part of the process—i.e., the discoveries of the student himself—is lost or impaired. This is a set principle which, after years of working with groups, I myself can only partly follow, but which I find I follow more and more each year. And I can observe it constantly in my teacher and colleague, Charlotte.

8 WHO IS STANDING?

I doubt if we ever stand naturally until we begin to recover the awakeness and wholeness that we had as little children, before we were taught about the "right ways" and the "wrong ways." Certain it is that most of us, most of the time, avoid standing at all, and generally speaking this gets truer as we get older. But I am very aware of changes in my own sense of standing over the years, in which, thanks to this work, my standing at age sixty is closer to what it was at six than perhaps at any age in between.

I well remember catching my first trout at age six, in a creek on the California coast near where I am writing now. One had to wait for them to bite, and this waiting was naturally done standing, the position of greatest alertness for fishing and best permitting response. I spent hours in what I seem to remember as full attention to the ever-present possibility of sudden action just out of sight in the deep pools or rippling currents. It seemed pure pleasure to me. No doubt that is why I relish the scent of nettles and bay leaves to this day.

But such special stimuli are not essential. What healthy child, out of school, does not spend half his life standing? Whether it is the life of the country or the life of the city makes little difference. Erect, one sees more; erect, one can be anywhere; erect, one is ready for whatever happens. Only babies cannot stand. Only grownups get tired standing.

Soon, however, other elements appeared. I was short. Mother was always measuring my height. Had I been tall for my age, I should no doubt have been constantly reminded of that. Gradually the comparison between myself and others came to be a regular corollary of standing. Furthermore, certain memorable moments of standing were moments of trial by my superiors, in school and at home; it was useless to "stand up" to them and actually more fitting to slouch. On the other hand, whenever these superiors took notice of my standing, it was to tell me to stand up straight and look them in the eye—something I had always done quite naturally until I learned what an avenue of aggression the eyes could be and how dangerous it was to meet that aggression and appear "impertinent."

I heard much, in those days, of broad shoulders and deep chests. This also became a half-conscious consideration in standing, for I think it never occurred to me that chest and shoulders also existed in sitting—which, in Mother's eyes, seemed mainly a function of the presence or absence of "backbone." Luckily, I was not a girl; it seems to me I would not have stood at all had I also been burdened with the cloud of ambiguities with which my world surrounded the advent of "curves."

Standing also involved my hands. Since the pants I wore had pockets, my hands were often in them: occasionally just to keep warm, but more often to toy with something in the pockets, a coin or a marble or a knife, or perhaps with my genitals, or just because it seemed safe and cozy there. In any case, this offended my superiors, who required me, in addition to standing straight and looking them in the eye, to take my hands out of my pockets. Had such encounters truly been an invitation to my full presence, as was the encounter of God and Moses on Mount Sinai, I am sure all this would have happened by itself without being asked for. But such divinity was absent. After the ordeal, there would be an escape, and part of the natural reaction would be to slump a little more than otherwise, look devious, and keep both hands firmly in my pockets, whether there was anything there or not.

Like everyone, I was once in a while cuffed or slapped by someone bigger than I. Gradually this experience joined the other elements present in standing that determined the where-abouts of my head and the degree of tension in my neck. This was also a prime question in any wrestling or scuffling, and in almost every case when any fist or missile was aimed at me. Ducking came naturally and developed into a useful and satisfying art; but some of my friends who had to duck too often never afterward lost the sense of danger quite enough to let their heads stand free.

What soon came too was a whole spectrum of *images*, from books, movies, and everyday talk, prescribing where and how the head should be in a variety of circumstances. Heroes held their heads high and erect; cowards cowered; the villain in action looked furtively, with head drawn close to protecting shoulders, and in capture stood with his head hung in shame; the pious lowered their gaze from a sinful world, or looked up to their maker in supplication. For every condition, it seemed, there was a right way for the head to be, especially in standing, and by this one could judge others and be judged.

There was also the question of vigilance. I was not born with a knowledge of the many hazards in the world, and I suppose I was often saved from unexpected collisions by the warning, "Look out!" For a child, whose attention is naturally drawn to details of life before he has any experience of what may be in the background, such warnings may be vital. But the child soon learns by himself that a background with potential dangers is often present, and then the continued admonitions to keep one's eyes open and be on the watch simply lead to a generalized distraction and anxiety. Probably English produces even more difficulties in this respect than the *Achtung!*, *attention!*, or *¡cuidado!* of other European languages, which have a less specific appeal to the eyes, even when the affective communication is the same. And probably the worst of these is the common American mode *Watch yourself!*

However that may be, in addition to being on the watch for trouble, I was soon watching myself much of the time and conscious that God might possibly be watching me, too. When my mother told me that she could tell by my eyes when my young friends and I had been "playing with ourselves," the circle was complete, and henceforth my own eyes stood guard over themselves.

Definitively, from that time on my standing was self-conscious. But *self-conscious* standing is not the same as *conscious* standing. In the sense of the word that I am trying to develop, it is not standing at all. It is a reaction, not to the pertinent realities of one's own inner structure and living needs, but to the real or supposed judgments of others, either actually present or remembered in the past. It is the core of stage fright and of our frequent queasiness about being photographed.

It is thus that work on conscious standing, or arriving at the point where the felt realities outweigh the imagined opinions, can be as truly a work on coming to oneself as is the long and, for the beginning, arduous sitting in *zazen*.[1]

I think my most vivid experience of standing, which for a moment wiped out the effects of years of conditioning, occurred shortly after my twenty-first birthday when I found myself in an expensive mental "retreat." I had been agonizing for months about what I felt was my essential dishonesty, and I had reached a point where I felt anything I said about myself was false. Not unnaturally, this was interpreted as an inclination to suicide.

The approaches of the psychiatrist in attendance seemed irrelevant to my difficulties, and since I felt an added guilt in accepting the luxuries of the place I decided to leave. This appeared to present no problem, since my private attendant had been too uninterested to keep up with me and I had been free to walk in the countryside as far and long as I chose each day. But when I finally told him I was going to get a bicycle and take off, he was jolted awake, and the next day I was taken to a real retreat with locks on the doors. Since I was no longer a minor, I could be admitted only with my own consent or by an act of committal. My whole struggle had been with my own negativity, but when the papers were laid on the table and I was asked to sign them, it was with a fully positive sense that I said, "*No!*"

I still thrill at the memory. We had been seated. When I rose now, I rose a free man. The fact that I was being incarcerated seemed incidental. The next evening, when the attendants

1. See Appendix B.

were at supper, I dropped my overcoat and shoes through the few inches that could be opened in the hospital window, squeezed myself through a square ventilator I had discovered eight feet above the lawn, and was free, outwardly as well as inwardly. I had secreted a twenty-dollar bill as I was being processed for admission; and in no time I was on a bus headed out of the state and on the first leg of my way to a lonely island that I had read about, where a new period of growth was to begin for me after my long self-repression.

My first act after this declaration of independence had been to come to standing. Authority was *there*, as it had always been, but now *I* was *here*. I could feel it from head to foot. Whatever I might lose from now on, I would at least not lose the taste of full presence.

Both before and after this event, there were many moments when life, so to say, brought me to myself—moments in love, moments in facing responsibilities and challenges, moments of full response to situations in which the consciousness of direct reality overshadowed consciousness of the past and apprehension for the future.

But it was to be many, many years before I would begin to work systematically to recover this possibility of presence which a single clarification of circumstances had once brought me to.

9 STANDING, FROM FOOT TO HEAD

Though standing is not standing, as I mean it, except when it is a unitary activity of the entire person, we can nevertheless work on it from any one of a number of approaches. One, very naturally, is through those complex elaborations of the organism nearest the ground—what we call "feet"—which have evolved specifically for the many activities which directly involve our reliance on the support of the earth. At the center of these activities is standing. On one side of standing, so to speak, are the practical activities, such as running and fighting; on the other side is dance. Really to stand can have the same relation to any such activity as a single sustained note on a flute or violin can have to a sonata. As our lips are to the flute, or our fingers to the violin, our feet are to the earth.

Of all human forms of celebration, I suppose dance is the most ancient and universal. It explores and glorifies the prime human and animal capacity of movement throughout the entire organism. As a way of becoming attuned to the mobility in others, and of sharing vitality, it has no equal. But it does not even require others. I have more than once spent the night dancing by myself. Even in solitude, it can have unparalleled meaning, as in the allusions of Don Juan, in Carlos Castaneda's books, to the warrior's last dance, when death itself must sit by, waiting until the dance is over.

But for most of us life is not a dance. We think nothing of committing our feet to imprisonment in shoes, and even blame them afterward for the consequent feeling that they are "killing" us. Many of us quite literally consider our feet inferior and "beneath us," and are horrified at the thought of entering a formal room barefooted, as we do barehanded.[1]

Two incidents from my life in New York throw a strong light on attitudes toward the feet. Once, when Charlotte and I opened our studio for a tenants' business meeting, about a third of our neighbors declined to enter because we asked them, for the sake of the studio carpet, to remove their shoes. But in another "studio"—an ancient industrial loft with ragged splinters in each board of the floor—where a drummer I knew held public calypso dances for a living, young people came for a thrill they could not find elsewhere. To dance calypso with shoes on would be like swimming with shoes on. I asked, "How can you manage with such a floor? Don't they get splinters?" "Oh they do," he answered, "and they love every one of them."

In the classes, we need not resort to splinters to wake up our feet. When anything brings them more to our attention, if we *allow* the attention, changes in their functioning may occur spontaneously, and such changes will always be toward the more appropriate. Nevertheless, it is unlikely that we are conscious of anything more than the vaguest sensation of the structure and function of the feet, even if we know the names of the bones and anatomical divisions and have a picture of it all in our mind from the anatomy book.

One thing we can easily do to make good for this lack is to sit down and explore our feet directly. With our own hands we may go deeply into them, discovering and enlivening the many joints and ligaments of which a foot consists. How far and deep must one go to follow the identity of a given toe until it becomes lost in the interior? What can we feel of the architecture of the arch? How does the heel seem to our palm and our fingers, in its aspect as bone and its aspect as padding?[2]

Of course, we may equally explore the foot of a partner. This,

1. The opposite is true in Zen practice, as was also the case on Mount Horeb—see Exodus 3:5.
2. If, at any time in reading this book, the reader should find it becoming abstract and remote and requiring effort to follow, I urge him to remove a shoe and spend five minutes exploring his own foot. Afterward, if he really wants to get up and take a walk, he will do so; but if he wants to read, I promise it will become easier for him.

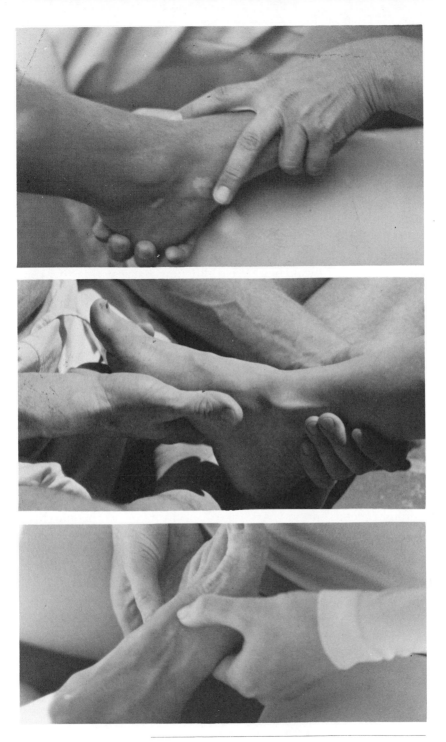

We may equally explore the foot of a partner.

in a new group, can create some tense moments. For who has held the foot of a stranger in his hand and worked with it dispassionately? Can there be such friendliness? Indeed, who has touched the foot even of a loved one without soothing, massaging, caressing, or simply playing with it? Few of us are able simply and genuinely to explore, as we did in childhood before we were warned not to, and as we are asked to do now—especially when the exploration is not just on the surface, as with a sculpture, or mechanical, as with the moving parts of an anatomy model. When exploration is really deep and felt, very much becomes awakened. We shall now harvest this awakening as we come back to standing.

Once again we take time to feel where the floor is. How do we relate to it? Let us close our eyes again: it may be easier this time. Many people now feel that they *are* relating to the floor. They no longer stand on their feet but on something which they feel really supports them from below. The feet feel flexible and alive, not stood on but free to explore what they touch, as the hands a moment ago were exploring them. Already the faces of the group may show the pleasure of this extension of consciousness to hitherto deprived regions. Perhaps we, too, have hands down there, as do our cousins the apes.

Now the leader may ask, "Do you allow the connection with the floor upward into you?" And a little later, "Do you allow it through your knees?" Afterward, a number of people may well report that they found their knees were locked. When they gave up this locking, readjustments could be felt taking place in the ankles or the pelvis or higher.

We may proceed upward in all sorts of ways in this question of allowing a fuller, more organic connection with what we stand on. For instance, how high above the floor is the pelvis? As thighs and calves wake up,[3] slight changes may occur

3. At some point the reader may become disturbed by an unfamiliar use of metaphor that characterizes what is certainly always in danger of becoming a "sensory-awareness jargon." New bottles are needed for our new wine—if such it is, as it seems to me. But until these new bottles arise from the communicative genius of a whole people, we in this work must use familiar words in unfamiliar connections with the hope and steadfast intention of not creating one more "trade" language.

spontaneously. Or we may deliberately tighten our buttocks or our stomach muscles, taking time to notice how this affects our relation to the support under us, and noticing the changes as we gradually give up the constriction to allow more connection through. Reports often follow of an opening, resulting in a sense of contact with the floor throughout the organism. Changes may be felt as far away as in neck, eyes, and lips, together with an increased sense of standing altogether, which is no longer just a gap in living but is now becoming a positive activity. Very often breathing changes, as one release triggers another, or perhaps sets up a constriction somewhere else.

Such deliberate tensing of muscle constellations, when followed by a very gentle and conscious release—quite different from the nerveless "letting go" so often practiced for relaxation —can be very valuable in bringing habitual contractions to consciousness, where they may slowly dissolve as the vital processes which they are inhibiting begin to be felt and permitted. This requires a fresh and new exploration on each occasion, as opposed to the technique or exercise which is repeated always with the same objective in view. For we are working not with ideas, but with consciousness itself.

Still standing, let us bring our hands gently to resting on the top of our heads. Through palms and fingers we can feel, if we are sensitive, not only our hair but also the temperature and perhaps the animation of living tissue underneath. This is as far up as we extend, just as the soles of our feet delimit our extension downward. What is alive in between? Is there some sense of our existing altogether between the meeting of hands and scalp at the top and of soles and floor at the bottom?

Somewhere in this extent air enters, penetrates to a constantly varying distance, and leaves; weight is passed on from bone to bone and muscle to muscle; fluids circulate; metabolic processes generate ever-changing energies. Everywhere sensory nerves are interwoven and there is the possibility of more awakeness. Our standing is an endless readjustment of these happenings to one another, depending on the clear functioning of our proprioceptive nervous system and on the flexibility of our musculature. It is impossible to practice with this too often.

In such trips through one's interior there is always a likelihood of getting stalled; so many toll gates and barricades have been set up over the years. Now and then, however, a new path opens: sensation and energy flood through; consciousness expands to regions heretofore out of bounds. One has a new and full recognition: I am alive there too! I exist: and I am standing on something which exists also.

The reader who is interested in such experimentation may feel like trying it out deliberately as I describe it. This is fine, if he has the time and patience. Otherwise, I would suggest waiting for some occasion when he is obliged to stand anyway. There are bound to be plenty of them. Perhaps he is waiting in line at the bank or in the supermarket, or for a bus, or standing in the subway or at a cocktail party. Instead of allowing his energies to sour into impatience or boredom, he may channel them into some such experiments as the above. He does exactly what feels agreeable and interesting, merely making the decision to forgo his customary inertia and to give himself, as fully as is practical, to exploration. He may explore anything that occurs to him. The only condition is that he give it his respect and time. If he can explore without hopes or expectations, but with the same kind of care he might give to doodling at the telephone, something will come of it.

10 WALKING: LOCOMOTION AND BEING

There is a little book by E. H. Shattock describing his stay in the Buddhist meditation center in Rangoon.[1] For some sixteen hours a day, in solitude, he practiced keeping his attention on his breathing, as evidenced by the rhythmic rise and fall of his belly. Every thirty minutes this meditation was varied with the experience of walking down the corridor, in which full attention had to be given to the alternate raising of each knee and the consequent swinging forward and descent to the floor of each foot. Such meditation is pure sensory awareness. Except for its exact structuring and rigorous discipline, it could fit into our work as a stream into a pond. There is none of us in this work whose practice would not be deepened and enriched by it.

The *kinhin* in *zazen*,[2] a five or ten-minute interval of meditative walking between thirty or forty-minute periods of sitting, is, however, closer to our normal experimenting. In the Soto form, steps are taken exceedingly slowly, and to maintain a full ease and balance is an art in itself. By the same token, to see the bare feet of a practiced Japanese priest meet and leave the floor in *kinhin* is more exciting to me than watching the footsteps of a panther.

Unlike standing, walking is so interwoven with every aspect of daily living that it is very often the first activity in which students notice changes and make discoveries. Usually this has to do simply with feeling what one walks on. But as time goes on, the whole process of locomotion, or transferring weight

1. Admiral E. H. Shattock, *An Experiment in Mindfulness* (New York: E. P. Dutton, 1960; Samuel Weiser, 1970).
2. See Appendix B.

from one leg to the other in order to proceed over the face of the earth, begins to regain some of the interest and liveliness which it has for young children and which has always made it a favorite occupation of nature-lovers and meditators.

In the studio, we may begin with just shifting our weight from side to side, slowly enough to feel how it is received and allowed down through our structure to the floor. Does the foot actually *give* the weight to the support below, or is it merely

The interest and liveliness which it has for young children.

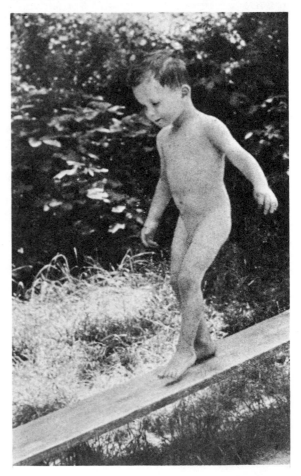

passive as the weight goes through it? Does the knee, and still more the hip, just receive and pass on weight as a chair does when we sit on it, or do these joints come actively into play with a sensitive coming to life of all the muscles that invest them? And the entire leg that is for a moment freed of weight: does it allow itself to be refreshed in that moment, or does it rather cling to the attitude of working? In a nutshell, this last is the whole great question of living in the present.

We may work for some time on treading, or shifting weight. As it more and more comes to gain our attention and interest, it may begin to resemble the day-long or night-long ritual of many age-old human dances. Were it to involve us more fully, so that knees, hips, pelvis, and lower back began savoring the elaborate transfer of weight from side to side, and trunk, arms, neck, and head began feeling, permitting, and glorying in their ever-responding balance, to the point of rapture through the entire organism, we should be led into those beautiful Caribbean dances, the Dominican *merengue* and the Haitian *méringue*. From foot to head, these are indeed nothing but a sort of fully felt, rhythmic walk in place, when reactivity in every joint maintains balance and presence over the full range from minimal to maximal movement. In such dances, I have seen couples in their seventies abandoned to the sensation of their own rhythmic shifting and redistribution of weight for twenty minutes at a time.

In our studio we do not use rhythms and we are not working at dance, but we do study to sense spontaneous readjustments of weight and balance as, first with one leg and then with the other, we come consciously to the floor in every variation of our weight. Animals are distinguished by the movement of their limbs away from and back to the supporting earth—movement comparable to the rhythmic, if irregular, movements of breathing. Perhaps this is one reason why Zen practice alternates sitting with *kinhin*, and why it can be so fascinating at the zoo to see a bear or elephant walk, where such great weight goes hand in hand with such delicacy. Indeed, there is no reason we cannot find the same fascination in our own walking. It needs only to be more fully felt and lived.

It can well be imagined that this kind of work demands full alertness and much time. One cannot hurry through it. And yet the precision and total presence we work toward may be seen in the very swiftest movements of animals. Who, in the country, has not seen a hummingbird, poised at a honeysuckle, dart instantly and faultlessly to another, twenty feet away? Whether you watch a cat leaping from the floor and landing on a shelf or a quarter-ton gorilla swinging from a rope to a platform, you will see, if you look closely, that each limb comes to easy and utter readiness exactly when it is needed, and not a moment before or after.

It is always the same question: am I, as total organism, awake and reactive? Are my limbs merely my property, which I must regulate and guide, or are they *me*?

When we have explored these questions long enough, it can become a matter equally of interest and of delight that it is possible to leave behind our concern merely with "getting somewhere" and can now begin to *feel how we go*. Whether we get there or not, we exist on the way. Instead of pushing or dragging ourselves along, we *walk*. In the exhilaration of the actual coming to life of our legs, we can feel how dance must have originated. From our pelvis to the soles of our feet we begin reaching down to touch the earth, as from the level of our heart we might reach a hand out to a friend. And from where we touch the earth, our whole precarious structure, which we can so easily diminish, finds its height and breadth and freedom in motion as it can in rest.

Once, in the Zen monastery in Tassajara, Charlotte asked an old friend how long she planned to stay. "Until I can simply walk down this road," was the answer. "But you do," Charlotte said. "No," she answered, "when I am not concerned any more about what I have done or what I still have to do, not concerned with how I walk this road—when I can simply *walk* it." The friend had already been walking there a year.

11 HARA

As we practice shifting weight, we may find that the floor has performed the same service for our feet that a partner did for them with his hands. They may feel worked through and greatly enlivened. If so, coming back to simple standing will be a vivid experience too.

If, in standing, we now bring one hand to the lower back and the other to the belly opposite, something may immediately become apparent. The situation we have been exploring through feet and legs has at this level changed markedly. No longer are we a skeletal structure, more or less equally enveloped and intertwined with nerves and muscles. We are entirely different, front and back. Under the hand in front is *belly*: an envelope of muscles containing a vague and inarticulate mass, whose very name is embarrassing to a great number of people. We have been told that there are many vital organs in there, mostly having to do with functions that are still not quite mentionable in company, so that some of us remain faintly ashamed of them and have a tendency to pull them in a little farther out of sight than they are already. Indeed, this also seems prudent since they are not protected with bones like our upper torso. We have forgotten that this is the *hara*,[1] or seat of vitality, of the Japanese, the "wheat field set about with lilies" of the Bible, and the "guts" of our own vernacular.

Under the other hand, in back, we find quite different territory, distinct and solid, bone and muscle. Nothing to be ashamed of here. It is with this that we stand erect.

1. See also the book on this subject by Karlfried von Durckheim: *Hara, The Vital Center of Man* (New York: Fernhill, 1970).

But let us explore movement here. If we again shift weight from side to side, we can clearly feel these muscles coming into play, governing the masses above. Like the shrouds of a ship's mast, they respond to every rock and pitch. Is that a mast we have? Let us try something else. First let us come to quiet standing and then gently explore what may be movable a little lower, in hip joints and pelvis. Perhaps we roll the pelvis backward and forward—the specific movements of sexual intercourse. Sideways, movement is complicated by our standing, but back and forth the beautifully lubricated hip joints offer no resistance. But the hip joints do not move in isolation. As we give careful attention, our hand clearly feels other joints coming into play—in the sacrum, in the lowest vertebrae of our spine, and upward.

This could be an important moment. How many of us, men and women both, have relied since childhood on this region to hold us firm against the pressures of living: not our back bones, but our *backbone*, the mainstay of our character, a rock against force from without and against tenderness and yielding from within? And how many others, giving up the struggle, have allowed dead weight to slump down on these vertebrae and overwhelm their natural mobility?

Let us raise and lower our two enclosing hands, exploring how far up and down our back movement is possible. Once we begin such an exploration, we may get a taste for it and wish to try it over and over. Even when we remove our hands we can feel the movement.

Now let us bring our hands back and attend to the belly. What is happening here? Beneath our clothes we feel it, still a little vague, somewhat soft, somewhat hard. There are muscles here too, but not such clearly conscious ones. What were they doing while we were moving our back, or now that we are again standing still? Perhaps our hand becomes interested. Instead of merely holding the belly, it begins to open for it. The wrist softens, the palm and fingers give up imposing their shape and seek the belly's shape. And the belly responds to the now sensitive hand. It becomes alive. It gives up the holding back or pushing out and seeks its own shape, which the hand also seeks—rounded, firm but soft, movable, at the center of the moving organism.

Something has come to life here. Breathing has changed. It has become spontaneous. Between our hands we feel it, entering sensitively, finding its own way, perhaps penetrating and awaking secret regions long closed to awareness. Like the incoming and outgoing tide, this breathing is patient and ambitionless, bringing sweetness to whatever opens for it, insisting on nothing. Deep inside us, as tissues awaken, neighboring tissues stir toward more awakeness too. Consciousness is contagious.

And now, through the gentle workings of breathing, it may be that we sense back and belly changing together, freely and in balance—no longer active and passive, defined and formless. We begin to experience ourselves as a single organism, where everywhere are needs and everywhere faculties, with numberless interconnections to permit adjustments as the needs are felt. And we may find that anxieties ease, inhibitions weaken, as they are undermined by the warmth and life which so often follow hand in hand with consciousness.

Such an experience may come at any time in the work. One who has had the good fortune to be ripe for it, and the patience to allow it, will, I think, have learned something of the nature of love, and something of *hara*.

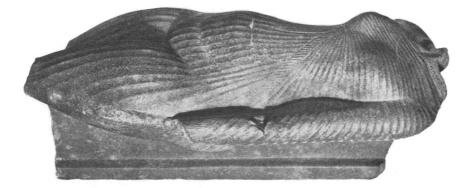

12 FINDING OUR STATURE

Most statues in the Western world, other than the military, are of figures standing; and in the statuary of ancient Greece and Rome almost everyone stood. One can equally come to one's full stature in sitting, as both Buddhist sculptures and Buddhist practice attest. In ancient Egypt, the source of some of the most marvelous creations in sculpture, significant figures are almost equally sitting and standing.

Our work, too, is largely divided between these two activities and among the great number of activities that depend on them, as leaves depend on the stem from which they grow. But for our purposes, the division is hardly a basic one. The difference between standing and sitting, in the more precise sense of the word which we shall investigate later, lies almost entirely in the activity of the legs. In both cases head and trunk, or the totality of organs and organic functioning, are fully involved, either in discovering and coming to their own well-being, under the influence of gravity, air exchange, and the support below, or in obedience to the numberless inhibitive or distracting elements of one's conditioning. We work that we may gradually admit more of all these factors into consciousness, where conditioning begins to lose its grip on us and to dissolve, leaving room for the objective realities. These realities, far from dissolving in the light of consciousness, become ever clearer and stronger.

The first part of this book will end with a study of sitting, which is the mode in which most of us Americans now spend the greater part of our lives. In the meantime, very much of our work with standing will be equally pertinent as a study of what can breathe life into that wasteland which usually passes

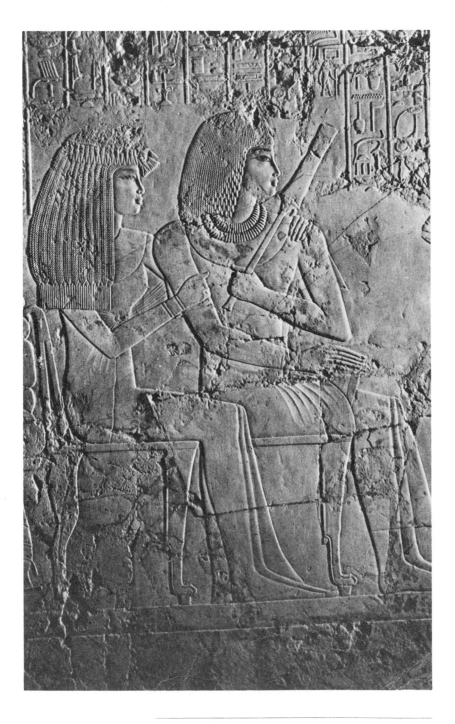

A study of what can breathe life into sitting.

among us for sitting, and of what brings such majesty and peace to the sitting figures of ancient Egypt and of both the ancient and modern worlds of Buddhism.

In the previous chapter I described an experience in which the hand, full as it usually is of the intent to mold and control, became interested in the nature of the belly and yielded to the magic of touch and discovery. This is, of course, especially possible for the hand, just as manipulation is, because of the many joints that allow it to adjust to such a variety of shapes. But few of us are at all conscious of the many joints in our spine. It is true we do not use our spine to mold and manipulate the world, as we do our hands, but we most certainly use it for yielding to or for resisting the natural and spontaneous movements of our own living.

It is the unique character of the spinal column that its many vertebrae make possible that union of flexibility with structure and gentleness with strength, which the great statues of the Orient represent. But the specialization of modern civilized man has brought a kind of premature arthritis to very many of us. In our loss of flexibility the most natural acts, like dancing and love-making, must often be performed by force of will. Force tends to rule our lives rather than strength, and letting go rather than yielding. But it is the tree that has nothing to let go and merely yields that displays such grace in the gale and has the resilience to survive.

Anything that can help sensitize the musculature and restore the natural mobility of our backs will do much to add to our sense of freedom and aliveness. A very simple and useful experiment to this end is that of coming from standing to a state of hanging over, in which the flexibility of the whole length of the spine becomes involved.

The elasticity of the adductor muscles of the legs is, of course, involved too. That is the reason for the popular calisthenic exercise of bending over and trying to touch one's toes, with which the experiment I suggest could easily be confused. But here we are not interested in how much we can stretch and how far we can get, but only in what happens on the way. If we go slowly and sensitively, we can feel constant inner changes as more and more of the musculature of legs and trunk yields to the downward pull of the earth, bringing about redistributions of mass and fluids in the inner spaces and new senses of weight and of extension. It is the extension of permissive tissues allowing their own weight to bring them gradually into an elasticity which feels very agreeable.

But as the back becomes more extended, the belly and inner organs are apt to become compressed, and circulation of blood to and from the head may be restricted. Such sensations can be most unpleasant. At the same time they are an unfailing

A state in which the flexibility of the whole length of the spine becomes involved.

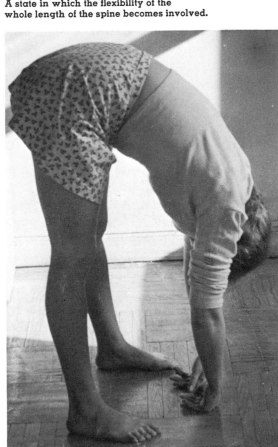

guide. One has only to return to where there is still a sense of ease and start sinking anew, more sensitive and alert, this time, to the changes that are called for—not only in trunk and legs but everywhere.

This gives the chance for very fine distinctions between achieving, allowing, and letting go. What is allowed feels good and right in itself; what is achieved feels good in spite of itself; what is let go simply feels limp and heavy. The allowing is when the person reacts as a totality; the achieving is when the person obliges himself, against his own resistance; the letting go is when he abdicates.

When it seems one is already hanging, there may still be developments if one sensitively feels out what slight changes may still be needed and granted to obtain more room for breathing and for circulation. These may lead to a finer balance between extension and compression, and to a more appropriate working together of the muscle systems with the complex inner organic functioning, so that one system of the organism is not performing at the expense of others. More giving is often possible, and more ease and well-being reached, when enough time is allowed.

But the real delight that may be found in this experiment is in the slow return from hanging to standing, when at last standing is not produced but *discovered*. It does not come at once. Many attempts may be needed before the subtle and often deeply rooted tendencies to effort can be sensed and abandoned. At first it may seem that one does not have the strength for it to happen by itself; one has to make efforts to produce it. At every stage on the way up, as on the way down, one may need to pause, go back a little to where it still feels easy and start rising anew—gradually feeling out in what phase of the process more energy is needed, or where this or that region is not fully involved in the activity and must be allowed to join in. It requires a strong interest, but offers rich rewards.

One may become lost and disheartened in one's own inner complexities. But when this happens, there is always a thread at hand to lead one out. At whatever point of the way between hanging and standing, one has only to give full attention to the facts of *breathing* and of *the floor*, and their power will do all the guiding needed.

After a while, one may become so fully alerted throughout that a fresh distribution of space and energy occurs which allows real inner freedom and a sense of total functioning. Then, when the work of rising is shared equally among all the tissues concerned, and is sustained by breathing and by the sure support beneath one, it can seem no work at all, but instead simply a yielding to one's own vitality, whose native energies tend naturally upward toward freedom and balance. As back and shoulders, belly, chest, and finally neck and head come gradually into what feel their right and natural relationships, allowing the inner channels to open easily for fluids and air, it seems like the response of a thirsty plant when given water, whose tissues fill until the whole organism stands erect and fresh. No penis or nipple, no sprouting seed rises with more totality and presence than does the whole person who has given full attention to the way from hanging to standing. It is then that standing can seem the full and natural expression of being.

Another frequently made discovery, as vertebra after vertebra and mass after mass finds its rightful place in the general unfolding, is that the moment when one feels *now I am standing* is always new. One comes to the recognition that there is no "standing position" for a person in the sense that there is for a

The whole organism stands erect and fresh.

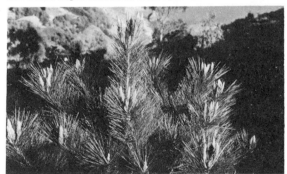

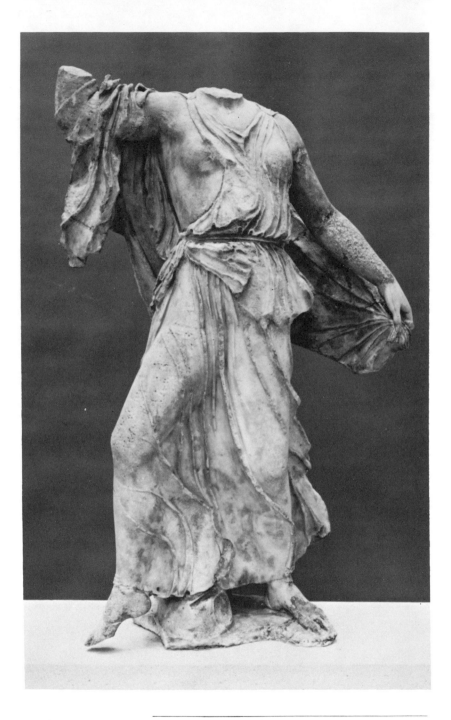

And left only the living being.

building. The positions that people assume, when not in reaction to a specific situation, are assumed in order to conform to some external model, or to some inner image or idea. The moment of arrival at standing, when we are occupied with our sensations, is never frozen into immobility or statuesqueness but remains in perpetual, subtle involuntary readjustment.

The sculptors of antiquity, in those enduring works where the ideational content is the least, cut away from their blocks of limestone and marble everything that might have landed in a fixed position and left only the living being. The same happens to each of us when our minds come to enough quiet so that we can sense our needs.

13 LYING AS AN ACTIVITY

In previous chapters, I have once or twice telescoped what might have been the fruit of many sessions into the form of a single continuing experience. It is seldom that such sequential expansions of consciousness take place at once. They may, of course—especially in the thrill of a first experience—and when they do, the person is filled with wonder.

But normally we travel along at an everyday pace. For most people at the beginning the attention span is short, and if they are not to wander off we must now and then shift direction. I believe this is the basic difference between our approach and that of *zazen*. There the student persists through thick and thin for the appointed time, hour after hour, despite all difficulties. Our work, which has a similar ultimate objective of full presence, takes a varying course, with many interruptions, changes, and times for rest.

What we use for resting is what most people unhesitatingly associate with resting: namely, *lying down*. And since we have only a floor to lie on, that is what we use—hoping, often vainly, that when people lie down they will neither get lost in daydreams nor fall asleep.

But it is by no means assured that in lying the student will either remain awake or come to rest, let alone both, regardless of the hardness or softness of what he lies on. So again and again, paradoxical as it may sound, we work on lying and resting itself. Indeed, we may remember that lying, which is the mode we have chosen for resting, is one of the "four dignities" of the old Chinese saying.

The reader, like the student, will almost certainly assume

that work on resting means practicing relaxation. I must state, however, that in certain vital respects it is the opposite. For most people's idea of "relaxation" is a kind of limpness, or what Charlotte often likens to a flat tire, or a flower without water, and this is what the practice of relaxation very often produces. We have heard too much of the "tensions of modern life" and have too little recollection of the marvelous tonicity of healthy living creatures—for instance, our own young children. So lying for us will be an *activity*, just as standing is. And as in all our activities, we will aim equally at inner openness for our own life processes and at sensitive contact with the environment. Whether this leads to more fatigue or to more refreshment is something each one can discover for himself.

We may start with a clearly practical question. Does everyone in the group feel he has room enough to lie comfortably? Even in a large room, many people in a group of beginners are so unconscious of space and so little in connection with the others that they will lie down helter-skelter anywhere, crowd-

The marvelous tonicity of healthy living creatures.

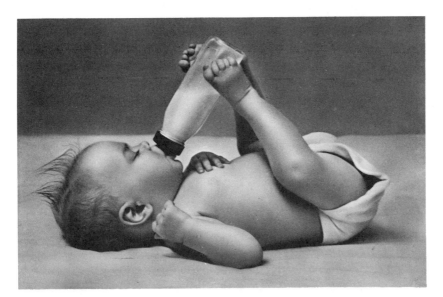

ing each other like so many weeds in a garden and leaving siz-
able open areas unused. It will not be possible to work this way
with any clarity. So we will ask specifically if everyone finds
he has enough room for both arms and both legs—so that the
air, for instance, is free to enter armpits and crotch, and
there is room for circulation of the blood.

A number of people may now shuffle here or there till they
can lie more freely. But a few may become conscious, if the
question is asked, that in spite of having plenty of room they
are nevertheless pressing their legs together, or pressing their
arms against their sides, or in some way pressing their head or
back against the floor.

If we ask them now not just to "let go" but to feel out carefully the difference between pressing and not pressing, they
may find that the pressing is not just a "tension" to be released
but has indeed a certain function. Crossed legs may feel lonely
and insecure when they come apart, or may tend to flop sideways. Tightly held arms may be giving one a feeling of protec-
tion. These are valid reasons deserving respect and should not
just be dumped in a compulsion to relax. Nevertheless, all this
is not resting. It consumes energy, even if not a great deal,
impedes circulation, and is in some sense a barrier between
the person and the floor under him.

Cautious experimentation in opening the arms and legs a
little may permit a certain flow of sensation that has not been
permitted before, and with it a flow of energy that changes the
way the limbs are lying—indeed the way the whole person is
lying—often bringing with it a new feeling of aliveness and
refreshment. This is something that would not have occurred
if the tension had just been mechanically relaxed, as with the
strings of a puppet.

Something very similar may be discovered if we raise one
leg or arm a little from the floor, stay to feel its weight, and let
it return. How does the surface feel on which we land? How
long does it take until we have fully arrived; and when we have
arrived, do we really allow resting?

Simple as this experiment sounds, it takes much practice for
most people to follow it through. We have been so trained in
exercises to strengthen muscles or to relax tensions, rather as

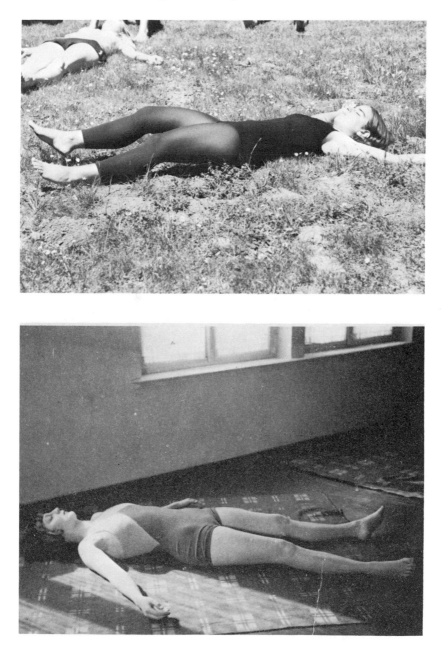

Raise one leg a little from the ground,
stay to feel its weight, and let it return.

The difference between just touching the floor
and coming fully to rest on it.

one might tighten or loosen the strings of an instrument, that we work on ourselves from the outside, so to speak, rather than from the inside. So much emphasis has been placed on the goals of our actions that we have lost the sense of what it is to be on the way, to approach and to *arrive*, as every pilot must when he lands his plane or brings his ship to dock. What we usually do is raise the leg, let it most of the way down, and then drop it, as we might a log on a woodpile and not as though we were concerned with living flesh and blood.

To make the experiment still clearer, we may ask people to raise the weight of the leg without leaving the floor at all, so they can feel the difference between just touching the floor and coming fully to rest on it. They are often amazed when they discover how far down one must allow the sinking in order to come to rest. Very frequently someone reports afterward that the leg in question seems to be lying deep in the floor, inches lower than the other one. This, of course, is the measure of the habitual withholding which has now been given up in one leg, but not yet in the other. Another person may announce the opposite: his leg feels light and floating, rather than sunken. This leg was previously heavy and lifeless and has now gained vitality. Such apparent contradictions merely illustrate the different habitual attitudes different people have acquired. I think no one, at any age, who makes such discoveries fails to be deeply impressed with them.

After a certain time of working this way, most people will feel the leg used has become more alive, longer, and, despite the energy employed, more rested than the other leg. Altogether they may feel greatly refreshed. In every sense, this could be called *work resting*.[1] What people usually mean by working is something like drawing water from a tank. One has a fixed amount of energy, and after a time the supply must be replenished. But this is like drawing water from a well, fed constantly by invisible springs. With each bucket drawn, the same amount flows up from deep in the earth, cooler and fresher than what was taken away.

1. *Rest Working* is the title of an interesting study in gland functioning by the Matthias Alexander student Gerald Stanley Lee, published in 1925 in Northampton, Massachusetts.

14 RESTING AS RELATING

What we have just explored in raising and lowering a leg while lying on the floor may equally be explored with arms or head. Many people have a persistent contraction in the neck—a pulling into their shell—which is usually acquired as my young friends and I acquired ours, as a childhood defense. In stressful situations this condition is aggravated, and even in lying it is not relinquished. This results in a sometimes painful pressure of the back of the head into the floor, which is not as compliant with our peculiarities as a soft mattress and pillow, but instead resists them steadfastly. Indeed, as Charlotte often points out and as we may soon discover for ourselves, the reason many of us awake from sleep more tired than when we went to bed is precisely because the soft beds we choose allow us to maintain our constrictions all night long.

A hard mattress, or, better still, the floor, makes many such constrictions unbearable and obliges one to give them up, at least while lying. Something has to give, and the floor will not. Willy-nilly, the circulation resumes its course and refreshment follows. During the first year of my study with Charlotte, I soon came to sleeping on a bare plywood panel, and, despite a few minor bruises, I never slept better. When two sleep together, if they love to sleep in one another's arms, such a surface may not be feasible; but even then it is well worth the trouble of experimenting how far in this direction two lovers can go. For the attitude of giving oneself is only enhanced when one gives to the environment.

To return to work: when raising and lowering the head while lying on the floor, it is certainly easier to use one's hands to help. This need in no way diminish the precision of the experiment. Working with the arms, however, is just like working with a leg, except that one may find it easier to raise only one leg at a time, but contrarily to raise both arms together. An interesting experiment is to compare the effects of moving both arms together and of raising and lowering them separately.

For many years as a carpenter I overworked my arms and shoulders. Millions who follow a single occupation have done the same. It is always a delight for me to lie on the floor and slightly raise and lower my arms, savoring the changes throughout these toughened regions where the roots of the arms disperse through the shoulder girdle as they begin to come awake for a present in which no achievements are asked, but only a readiness to yield outwardly to the support beneath and inwardly to the grateful play of breathing.

In this connection, I would urge the reader not only to try the same, but also sometime when he is in bed to experiment a little for himself in this familiar situation. Two external factors will then be present: the resistance of the mattress and the pull of gravity on limbs and covers. To raise any of the four limbs alone, or in any combination with another, may allow openings into the whole inner world. The only prerequisites are patience and interest in exploration, and the willingness neither to make an exercise of it nor to let thinking crowd out sensing. When these simple conditions are met, each movement has effects that may be felt through the entire organism. One may lie on one's back, on one's side, or on one's stomach; the differ-

Something has to give, and the floor will not.

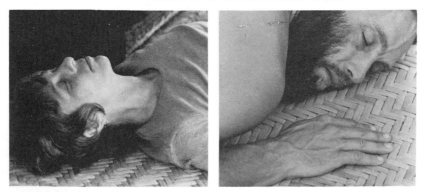

ent challenges, the different nuances in response, may become utterly absorbing. And as with every other occasion of giving complete, sustained attention to one's inner processes—which is the sense in which I use the word "meditation" in this book— the result is always refreshment rather than fatigue.

Even when lying with another person, one can experiment this way. Can one raise just enough of the weight of an arm or leg resting on the other so that it seems to him merely the sensitive refining of a connection? For that indeed is what it is. Then it cannot disturb him, but can only make his resting sweeter.

The reader may already have realized that in all these cases of how one may utilize a "rest" period of lying, whether on the floor, in bed, or on a meadow, the central element is how one relates to the environment. This is why we are so insistent that these experiments should not be regarded as exercises. What most of us mean by an exercise is something done for self-improvement according to this or that preconception or author-ity—often conducted in a sort of vacuum, in disregard of the environment, and leading one away from the real world and toward a narcissistic goal. Quite a different meaning, however, can be assigned to the word *practice*, which to me means sim-ply the opposite of theory. One exercises certain muscles in weight-lifting, in order to strengthen them. But one may *practice* weight-lifting to explore the activity or to discover how one relates to a given task. In this sense, one may exercise one's knowledge of French, as in the repetition of words or forms to fix them in memory, or one may practice it to gain the feel of another language and to communicate. Practice, thus understood, leads us out of the world of fantasy into the real environment. So, though I enjoy a little "exercise" as much as the next man, I find it important to emphasize that the word is thoroughly inappropriate to the activities I describe.

When we raise a leg and let it come back to the floor, it is not really different from drawing a bowstring and letting the arrow fly to the target. Thinking will not help us, nor will reading the instructions. We can only practice until we become more and more fully involved with the task. The bow has the power,

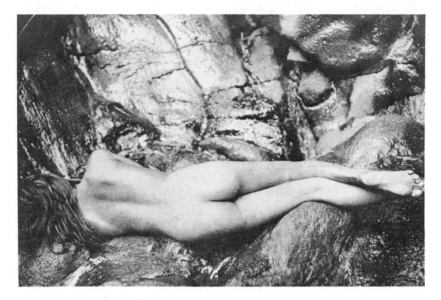

How one relates to the environment.

in our hands, to send the arrow to the bull's-eye. Herrigel spent six years in Japan studying archery until he could *let it happen.*[1] It may very well take us six years too, following our practice until we begin to feel through and through what we are doing, when we are with it, and when and where we are still uninterested or exaggerating.

Since we are not practicing Zen, we shall not work six years raising a leg. But in a sense, we do. In a sense everything we do is the same. This is again how our activities differ from exercises, which are always directed to particular goals, each distinct from the others. We are not interested in the healthy mind in a healthy body. We are interested in the total functioning person.

What we seek is to let ourselves be *with it*. As children, we naturally gave full attention to everything, though it all may have changed every moment. Then the authorities told us about our responsibility not just to do things but to do them *right*. Since

1. Eugen Herrigel: *Zen in the Art of Archery* (New York: Pantheon, 1953).

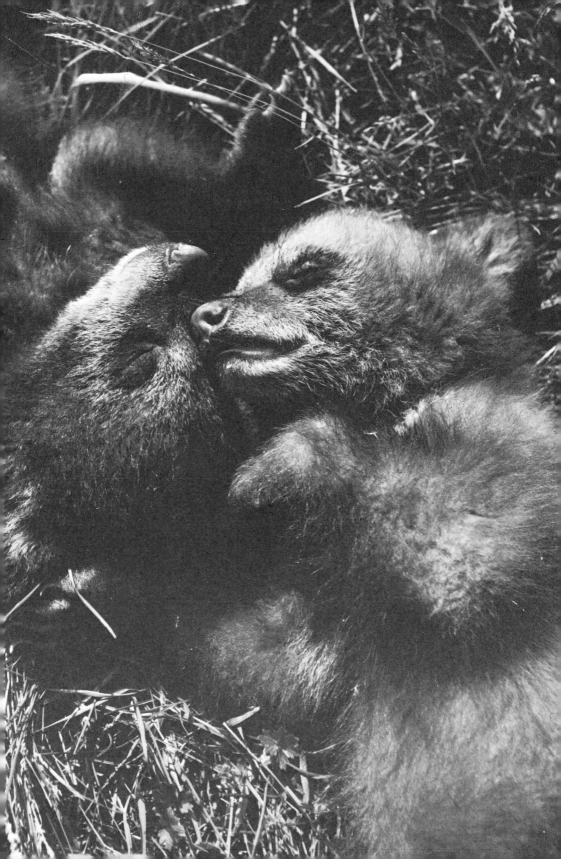

then, our attention has been divided between what we are doing and whether we are doing it right. Many of us became compulsive in our acts,[2] and many of us became resigned to failure; but that did not free our attention for the task. We are not able to give our attention fully; there are too many whispers of conscience distracting us. We must take the bull by the horns and deliberately practice, feeling how we do what we do, gradually learning to give up the cherished notions of the right way and the wrong way, which simply lead us away from the task itself, and coming more and more to feel the real situation and what it asks of us. Little by little we begin to get with what we do, now more, now less; and finally, perhaps, comes a spontaneous action, arising of itself from our full perception of the situation, when the arrow effortlessly hits the bull's-eye or the leg comes in full awakeness to the floor which offers it rest.

I cannot leave the subject of relating to the floor without touching on the delightful possibility we have here, too, of using lying to become more awake in our pelvis. For this we may enjoy experimenting at length (and the reader may equally enjoy experimenting) with raising our knees, while lying on our backs, and bringing both legs to standing with our feet on the floor. This changes the situation along the whole length of the spine, allowing the small of the back to come closer to the floor, and lengthening and opening the spinal musculature. The head will probably want to find a new and freer lying where the neck may also come more to resting.

Just bringing one leg at a time up to standing, or extending one leg after the other sensitively to its full length on the floor, offers so many opportunities for new discoveries in one's contact with the floor, and at the same time invites so many delicate readjustments in the pelvis, that one may remain engrossed in these activities for a long time. But perhaps the clearest experimenting can be done when both legs are standing precisely where they feel freest and strongest. If one then raises the pelvis very slightly, feels how one maintains it in the air and how this affects breathing, and then feels the way back

2. As in this report from a student: "All this week I have tried very hard to undo my overdoing."

to resting on the floor, there may be very interesting new sensations. The combination of the many joints between lower back and pelvis, and of the hip joints between pelvis and legs, together with the considerable weight involved, provides an unparalleled opportunity to sense what it is like when one allows a gradual settling down and a full coming to rest. One may never have dreamed that such subtle changes, or such clarity and delicacy of perception, could exist all through this vital region, from the lowest spine to the very depth of the groins.

Next to the head, this is the most crowded region of the organism. Our most powerful muscles make their connections here, next to our most delicate sensibilities. The great functions of reproduction and the vital necessities of elimination must find passage here, free and easy passage, like rivers among forests and mountains; and yet here we must have the strength to move our whole weight freely as we go about our affairs. No wonder that any refinement of consciousness in the pelvis, any reawakening of its natural sensitivity and mobility, will help us in a thousand ways. It will make sitting more distinct and real; standing, walking, and running easier; dancing livelier; love-making more sensitive. And any general

Both legs standing where they feel freest.

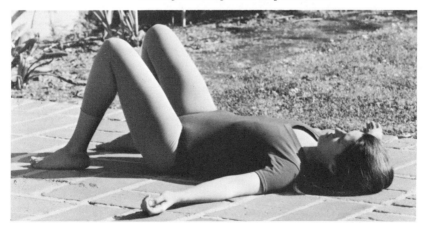

awakening and freedom of being at this end of us, which we sometimes wisely call our bottom, leads directly to a concomitant freedom and peace at the top.

■ Now that we have used it as a mode of working, and have explored some of its many actual components, lying can begin to become truly useful to us for its ostensible, but perhaps hitherto unrealized, purpose of offering rest.

In fact, of course, any change of activity may be restful. A vigorous game of tennis may be most refreshing after a day in the office, and reading an adventure story may be restful after a game of tennis. When I first worked as a carpenter in New York, where the union practices of the day claimed many heavy, unskilled jobs for carpenters which elsewhere were performed by "laborers," I would sometimes come home too exhausted even to think of going anywhere in the evening. But

---

A lying that permits the uninterrupted flow of metabolic process.

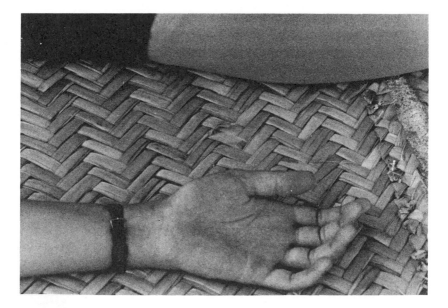

twice a week I would nevertheless drag myself into the subway and up to the classes in "modern primitive" dance at the Katherine Dunham studio. Here, where I first encountered Haitian and conga drums, and black forms in ancient ethnic movements, we responded to explosive rhythms with the speed and energy of dynamos. If one rolled on the floor, a puddle was left behind. Two hours later, I returned home, ready for bed it is true, but already as rested and refreshed as after a hot bath.

All this notwithstanding, sleep is the universal recourse from the fatigue that finally develops in all activities; and the active principle in sleep is a lying, mentally and muscularly quiet, that permits the uninterrupted flow of metabolic process. This, as we have found, is something that we can study, and at least to some extent arrive at, while awake. Now when we lie on the floor to rest between our different periods of experimentation, we can have some real hope of refreshment, and not of just being carried away by trains of thought.

15 SITTING

A good deal of our work takes place while sitting—with, and mostly without, chairs. But although we have a largely sedentary culture, this has not prepared people for sitting on ground or floor, as is the usual practice in many parts of the world, and as must have been the practice during the whole period of our evolution after our ancestors descended from the trees. Certainly there is nothing in it contrary to our natural structure. On festive occasions such as picnics and campfire gatherings, we take this primitive way of sitting for granted. Young people gathering around a guitar unhesitatingly prefer it to the use of chairs. Our babies sit like saplings, alert and effortless.

But many of us Western adults soon lose this faculty. We have created a physical scene that no longer requires it, and even in adolescence our thighs, pelvis, and back begin to lose their elasticity. When we sit on the floor, our ligaments, even our clothes, don't give; our backs and shoulders easily begin to ache; our ankles press; we clasp our knees, slump, or strain, and we must constantly shift. Of course, we are not very concerned: we have plenty of chairs. But the trouble is that when one loses the elasticity for sitting, it is lost for very many other things also.

These facts have been widely recognized, and there are many useful exercises one can try, especially those practiced in dance and yoga. But the stretches in dance are apt to be forced and not clearly felt, as is also true in yoga; and in yoga there is the added likelihood that one forms the habit of seeking and attaining rigid postures. One must not forget that yoga originated in a culture where everyone sat on the ground anyhow and great muscular flexibility was the norm. As its name indicates, it was a yoke, or restraint, a liberation not *for* movement but *from* movement, from the shifting sensory world to a union with the ideal. However diluted, some of this sense of achievement and self-control is still usual in yoga; and our yoga students, like our dancers, often find they have much to unlearn in order to come to a fresh and alive balance.

Nevertheless, every such exercise done patiently, in order to explore the changing limits of one's flexibility, rather than

Our babies sit like saplings.

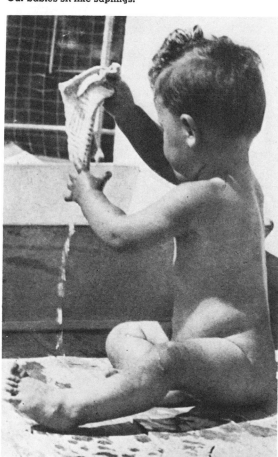

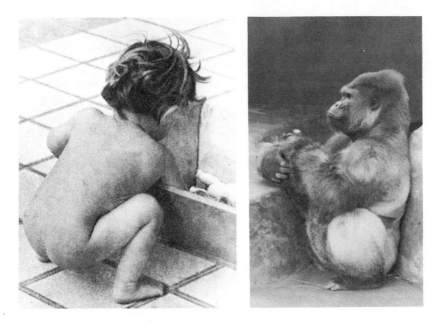

Among the world's squatters.

to attain a position, and done permissively and not with force, will be helpful.[1]

Exercises in flexibility are also less necessary in those cases, still common in many parts of the world, and with our own hikers and campers, where modern bathroom styles have not yet prevailed and where bowel movements are still performed as they were for our first hundred million years, namely in squatting. The *squattoir*, as I liked to call it, was one of my first vivid impressions of the grand old France of forty years ago; and the Japanese equivalent, without running water, I found equally impressive on our recent visit to Kyoto. It is hardly surprising that those most highly civilized people, the French and the Japanese, whose customs, at least until recently, have

1. It would not be fair to make these strictures on yoga without mentioning that in *zazen* also, in spite of the Zen (or at least Soto Zen) rejection of achievement as a goal, new students are taught exactly how to sit and what position to maintain. After a number of years, those who continue tend to become free and easy in it, and it loses its rigidity, as is undoubtedly the case with Indian yogis.

encouraged such flexibility and forthrightness at the exit of gastronomy, have been such masters at the entrance. And of course, among the world's squatters there is no laxative industry.

Nor is all this in the past. When I recently visited two New Mexico communes, I literally found some of the most exciting architecture in the toilets. With an obvious view of restoring good sense and dignity to these long-degraded functions, both had structures, exquisitely sensitive to light and space, equally divided between a Crane bowl and a simple hole in the floor. One at last had the freedom of choice: either to sit for evacuation on a seat, approximately as one sits for eating, or to discriminate between these processes like every dog and cat, and like Moses, Pericles, and Julius Caesar.

But in daily life we normally sit on chairs—or, better, *in* chairs. There is a great difference. It is instructive to visit a museum where a room of the seventeenth or eighteenth century is reproduced. All is for sitting *on*, with only a slight support offered to the back. Compare this with the Grand Rapids furniture of the last fifty years: the overstuffed chair and sofa designed to envelop rather than support, in which anything that could properly be called sitting is out of the question. It is the same with the Detroit car. When I recently drove a standard American car, my own Volkswagen bus not being available, I realized that no muscular activity was required of me other than the "fingertip (and toetip) control" advertised. In fact, the seat embraced me like a womb. I felt curled in the fetal position: ideally, I suppose, that of maximum comfort. Yet I was not comfortable at all. Why? I realized then that the designers had overlooked at least two major considerations. One: I had no umbilical cord and needed to breathe for myself, which in this position was possible only to a very limited degree. Two: the need for alertness and quick changes in response clearly distinguished life in the womb from life on the freeway. In this car, only the head and the extremities were expected to function, while all the rest of the person was considered just cargo.

One of the saddest consequences of this general alienation

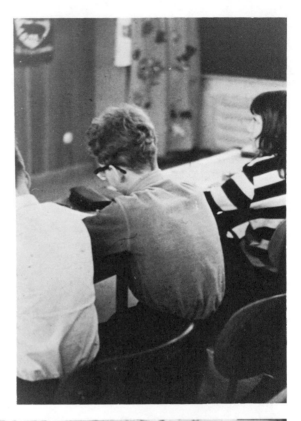

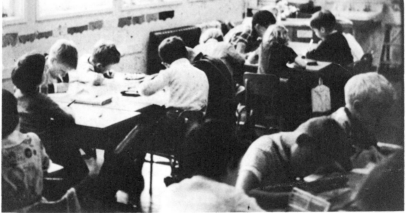

Long hours at desks.

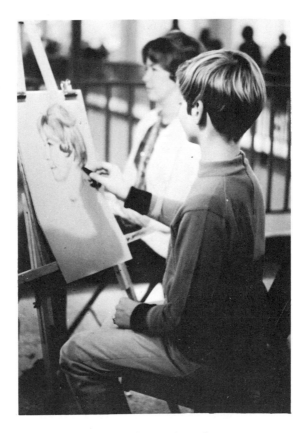

What a different sitting when one is awake
all through for the task.

from our real needs is the way we oblige our children to spend long hours at desks and in seats whose design has no relation to their organismic functioning. The accompanying photographs by Friedrich Everling[2] show some of the distortions and malfunctioning into which otherwise normal children are led for long periods in typical schools, affecting their vision, breathing, circulation, intellectual processes, and worst of all, their sense of freely existing as persons.

2. A student of Elsa Gindler's who has made experiments in combining classes in nuclear physics, of which he is professor, with classes in sensory awareness.

In our studio we have nothing but stools. Elsewhere, we try to have simple flat folding chairs available. We sit on them. The support they offer, like their shape, is perfectly distinct. We let our feet come consciously to the floor, avoid crossing our legs, and rest our backs against the backs of the chairs. This last, of course, is not possible with stools, and it gives us the opportunity for an interesting clarification. It will become apparent, if the question is raised, that sitting thus on the chair we are not simply sitting, but are also *leaning*. Part of our weight is supported vertically and part horizontally.

Granting attention, we can easily feel how much weight we give to the back of the chair. (Or does it feel more like *pressure*?) Could we say that we relate to it? We may leave the back of the chair, come to sitting with nothing behind us but air, and return, more alert and sensitive, to leaning. Are we also awake for the floor? More openness may have to be permitted in pelvis and legs before we have the sense of really coming down to the floor. We may experiment with very slightly raising and lowering our heels, or moving our knees, to become more conscious in the musculature connecting legs with trunk.

Now let us try coming to actual *sitting*. We leave the back of the chair for good, sensing the readjustments throughout our structure as the support is given up, feeling how we come more and more into the vertical, simultaneously reaching down to the seat of the chair and rising up from it.

If we are now really to relate to what we sit on, we must become much more awake than usual in the region of us directly in contact. Let us rise a little from the seat, pause, and gently find our way back without using hands or eyes. Can we find it? Ah! There is a definite meeting. Our nerves are as good down there as anywhere.

The question comes up: are we just padding down there where our sitting originates, as we may always have imagined? By no means! We begin to feel a definite structure, possibly as firm as the chair itself. To explore it let us raise one buttock and slip a hand underneath. Somewhat gingerly, we sit now on our own hand. Something in our bottom is not just firm but hard. Can we raise the other buttock, to sit on both hands at

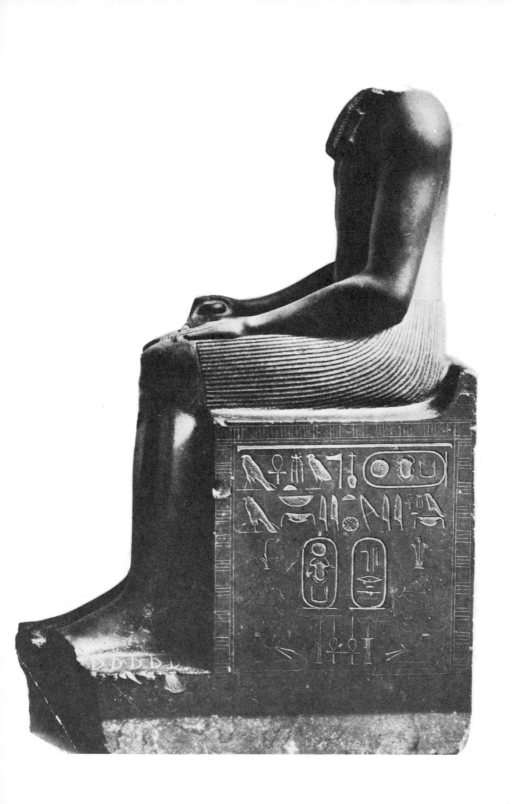

once? Ouch! We had not dreamed there would be such hardness. With relief, we divide our weight between our two hands, so as not to crush either. What is so hard in there? Even our heels do not seem so hard.

Cautiously, buttock by buttock, we leave our hands and return to the unprotesting seat. It becomes clear that, whatever the singular nomenclature for our bottom, sitting is actually divided between two sitting-bones. We can allow an equal or unequal distribution of weight, for more or less pressure on the seat, and of course on our own tissues. We can also "walk" with these sitting-bones. With a little experimentation, we find we can walk here and there on the seat till we are quite familiar with it, perhaps discovering a very agreeable perceptiveness in our own pelvis. Finally we may perch ourselves on the very edge of the chair, where our thighs no longer rest on anything, but bridge out into space. By this time our whole pelvis may be wide awake.

We have now found our architectural base, the sitting-bones. From here, if awake and free, our thighs openly extend, and our well-defined, clearly conscious legs come down to the floor. Our feet rest sensitively and at ease. A platform, which we call the chair, elevates the rest of us to about the level of our knees, but from there up nothing outside ourself supports us.

Again we may close our eyes for clearer sensing. What holds us up? Perhaps we hold ourselves up. Who has ever been told: *sit up straight?*

Let us sit up straight. Let us really hold ourselves erect. How does it feel? We need time to find out; it doesn't become clear all at once. Someone reports he feels tight in back and neck. Another finds his breathing shallow. Another says he feels like an image, not a person. We maintain the posture until it begins to be tiring and then, very slowly, allow changes for more ease.

After a while, an observer would notice that "ease" means quite different things to different people in the group. Some are still in a vertical sitting, others deeply slumped. We must explore further.

We are all asked to slump now. It should be without exaggeration, just what is familiar to us. How is it now? Perhaps quite

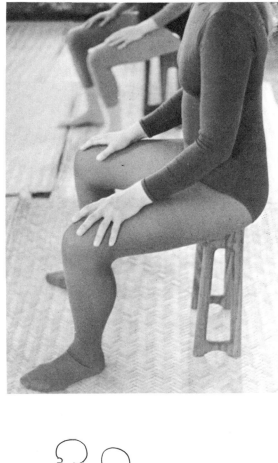

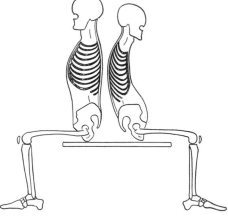

Our architectural base, the sitting-bones.

comfortable. It is, after all, what we believe to be "relaxed"; it has some of the familiarity and comfort of an old shoe.

But let us stay awhile: there is something unusual in this situation. We are not hearing a lecture; we are not eating at a lunch counter, where we always sit slumped, or watching television. We are not even collapsing from exhaustion. We are just sitting slumped to feel how it is.

Finally we are asked, "Who still finds it comfortable?" Only one or two hands are raised.

"What is not comfortable?"

There are many answers. "I can't breathe." "There's no room for my stomach." "My back hurts." "I feel constricted all over."

What changes would we have to allow *now* for more well-being in sitting? But gradually . . . let us sense where we go— not just change blindly, as we do so often. Where is more room needed inside for all that lives there? Not where do we *think we ought* to have more room, but where do we *feel it needed*?

Let us bring our hands to the top of our heads. Room is needed in the shoulder girdle too, especially if our hands are to rest lightly on our head, so that the head does not have to press up against the hands. How far is it, when we are not straining anywhere, but just awake and open, from our hands above our head to the seat below our sitting-bones? What may need room to live and breathe in between?

Subtle changes begin to occur in those seated: tentative readjustments, half-conscious inner gropings. How wide are we, when we allow our natural width, without stretching? How much space do we need from front to back? Is there any sense of life in our backs? How deep do we allow ourselves to be— down to our bottom, till we come to the seat?

To an onlooker, the faces would now be quiet as in sleep, the habitual expressions gone, eyelids still, but radiating a deep inner awakeness. No one is in his habit any longer, but is exploring something new. We let our hands find their way to rest now on our thighs, so that from the seat trunk and head rise freely as high as we go. Very striking: for the first time, perhaps, many hands *come to resting* on the thighs as butterflies on flowers, without at the last moment just dropping. Our

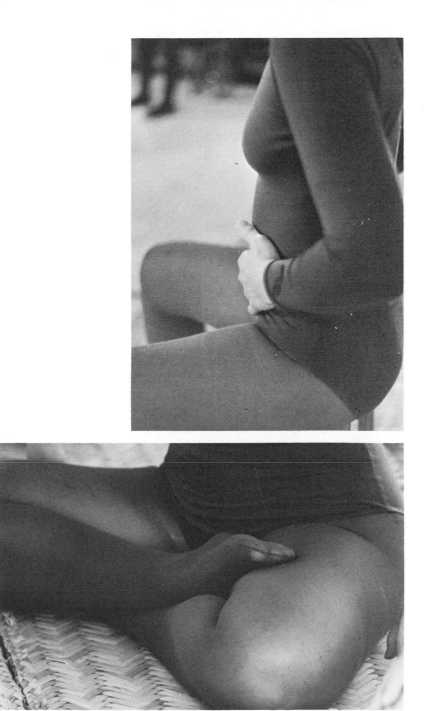

Where is room needed for all that lives there?

eyes open. On all sides, others of the group sit near us, like the flames of candles. Each of us feels it in himself. We are alive. We sit.

On other occasions we will work with partners, for there is no end to the work on sitting. One person sits on chair or stool; the other comes gently with his hands to back and front, finding the living person. Where is our inner living felt, where we need room for being? Hours can be filled with such explorations, to undo the work of the numberless hours of our lives that have been spent acquiring and consolidating the inhibiting habits. No time is too much, if we are with it. Only if we do it as exercises for an image of self-improvement does it become empty and fruitless.

Or we may slap and massage each other; dig with our fingers into the intercostal or the shoulder muscles to wake them up

Quiet as in sleep,
but radiating a deep inner awakeness.

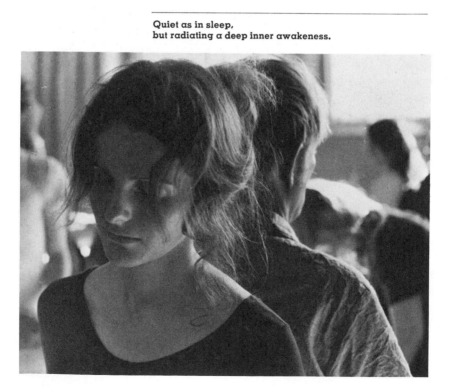

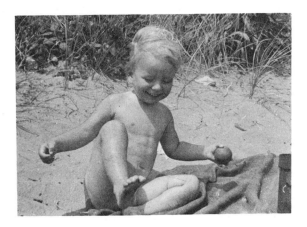

Closer to that marvelous sitting of young children, alive and effortless.

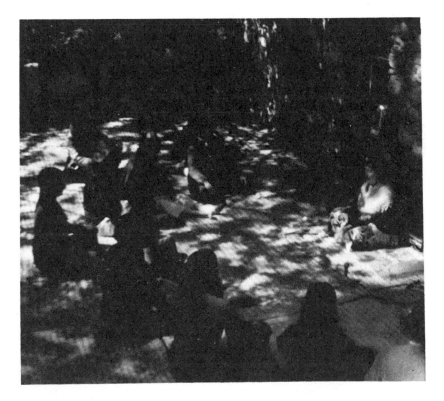

and stimulate their elasticity; work, specifically in sitting, to awaken head and eyes—for always here, in what Charlotte likes to call our "control tower," if peace and clarity come, more awakeness and freedom will tend to spread everywhere.

As it seems feasible, we will divide our work on sitting between chair and floor, for gradually, as we become more awake in our inner living, we will come closer to that marvelous sitting of young children, which we can see also in our zoos with the apes, where no furniture is needed at all, and we can exist in peace, alive and effortless, open for the light of our consciousness to burn according to its nature.

Toward
a More
Sensitive
Relating

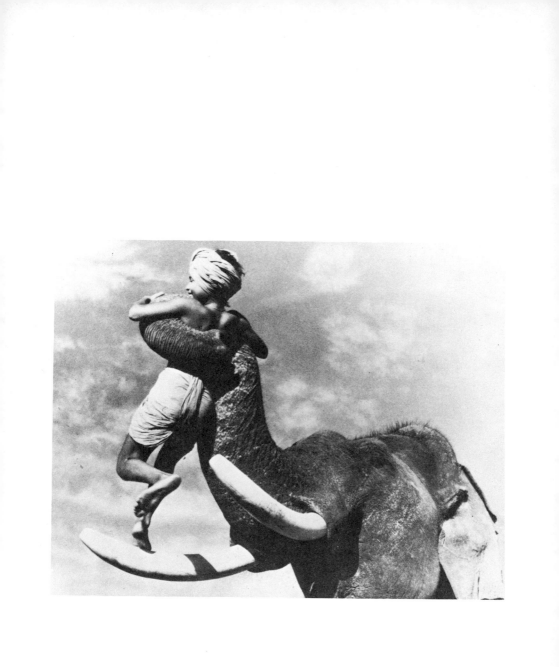

It is often said that we are born and die alone, but this is hardly true. The old Navajos, when they felt their time had come, did indeed ask to be escorted to some lonely place which they had chosen, where farewells were said and they were left alone to spend their final hours undisturbed, coming to peace with the surroundings. But this was in the full ripeness and at the very end of life. We are born very differently. No sooner have we left one human ambience than we seek another, exchanging the darkness, warmth, and quiet of the womb for the life on earth of crying out and seeking for the breast. It is in a primarily human environment that we spend our lives. Whether this human environment is felt as unique and separate from the general environment or merely as a special manifestation of it depends for most of us almost entirely on our culture. But our culture is in a way itself an environment, which each of us in minute ways is constantly modifying. How we modify our culture depends on the clarity with which we perceive it, and perceive *through* it, and on the sensitivity and integrity with which we relate to the individuals and objects without which no culture could exist.

16 SLAPPING AS A STIMULANT

Wild animals are kept in a constant state of sensory awareness by the mere facts of their environment—an environment for which the whole course of evolution has prepared their many faculties and which tends to keep these faculties in constant and well-balanced activity. We, however, as individuals in a highly organized society, are obliged to specialize. We become machine operators, or business executives, or lawyers, channeling our energies, often very narrowly, during our productive hours. Indeed, the more productive we become, the likelier it is that we have limited our general organismic functioning quite strictly to those areas which merely serve our social and economic roles.

The practice of sensory awareness would revolutionize all this. I do not mean the classes described here. But I *do* mean a quiet feeling through of whatever one undertakes. Just as we work in the classes with any activity that suggests itself, so in social and economic living there is no activity that cannot be performed either mechanically or with full attention and interest. One is not naturally a machine performing a task, whether the task is laying bricks or computing. Each of us represents anew the most highly evolved sensory and cognitive nervous organization in existence. That is why we like to watch birds and chipmunks. They have their way of living, and we have ours, and in both there can be such a thing as *joie de vivre* during the day, and the weariness after joyous labors that draws us all to rest at the end of it.

As things are, however, the weariness of a group of people assembled for a class of ours at the end of the day is in good part boredom, or the condition resulting, not from the overwork of certain faculties, but from the underwork of others. During the day, consciousness of the drain on one's vitality consequent on blocks and imbalances in functioning has been warded off by a steady intake of distractions: the radio, idle conversation, tobacco, chewing gum, and the like, and in the evening anesthesia is normally prolonged by the chatter of television. How difficult must it now be to forgo distractions and give attention to the muted and unfamiliar voices of one's own senses!

Resting on the floor often brings little relief from this type of weariness. A more effective tonic is stimulation. It is the same situation as the recess in school. The children have been cramped at their desks for an hour or so, compelled to focus attention on matters that often have not caught their interest, and for ten minutes they are allowed to run around in the school yard. Who does not know the shrieks and shouts, the bursts of energy surrounding any ball, any encounter, any game?

Our students need a little excitement too, to start the arteries pulsing, discharge the wastes, and renew the oxygen—in a word to get refreshed after the tedium of the day. If a bear should now push open the door and enter the room, fatigue would vanish. Then we might learn what energies develop when, as in a magnet, all our molecules point in one direction.

In fact, it is the gradual arrival at such a state, where everything in the organism works together, not aimed toward a bear but toward the central life process of breathing, which makes it possible for some people to sit in meditation day and night, without the usual need of sleep for restoration.

But we are neither practicing Buddhist meditation nor in a situation to rely on alarms and floods of adrenalin. What can we do—we who are here to come to quiet and to sensing?

One thing we can indeed do is to *slap*, either ourselves or others—not as a punishment, of course, but as a stimulant. Our entire surface is there to be aroused, a continuous network of nerve ends and blood vessels, all leading underneath and into the interior.

How we slap is something we shall have to study, just as we

found there is very much to study in how we lie. Most people can no more just start slapping themselves or another with any delicacy and discrimination than they can sit down and start playing the piano. Nevertheless, if the slapper is not actually bored, timid, or vindictive—and sometimes even if he is—what he does will awaken nerves and start the blood going wherever he slaps. So for better or worse, we may as well start right in and slap ourselves all over, with particular attention to any areas where waters may seem stagnant and tissues drowsy.

After a few seconds of slapping it may be wise to interrupt things so as to feel what we have done till now and how it goes on working in us. We might even recognize whether we are unheedingly punishing or comforting ourselves instead of waking ourselves up. It is astonishing to see the incredulity and amusement on people's faces, followed by growing interest and pleasure, when they are first introduced to this simple remedy for dullness.

When still more stimulation seems indicated, one person may stand with arms extended, or may hang over toward the floor, while another—or, better, two or three others—rain their attentions on him. In many cases pleasure now rapidly becomes delight, as the receiver finds himself bobbing among the slaps like a speck of cork in a glass of champagne.

How we slap is something we shall have to study.

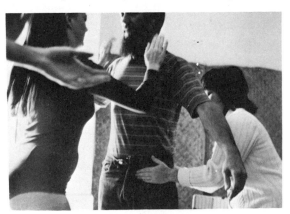

Since enthusiasm in such an activity comes easily and is naturally infectious, the leader may often have to caution against what may well sound and feel like beating, and remind the slappers, as well as those slapped, to permit their own breathing. Many people, when aroused, will attack another as they attack cold water at the beach, plunging in and splashing with breath held, so as to do as much, and feel as little, as possible. In such a case, consciously to permit one's own breathing brings immediate changes, for the stiffness in wrists, elbows, shoulders, neck, and head that prevents sensitive slapping (as well as reactivity to slapping) is hardly possible without the corresponding rigidity in chest and belly that inhibits breathing.

The study of slapping is a matter of coming awake for the nature and reactivity of what one slaps. We must become very present, to feel what we are doing. Since in our experience a slap has usually been a rebuff or a punishment, we must now give it special attention.

The slap which the adult administers to the child in anger is normally his reaction to some real or fancied threat in the child's action to himself or to what he values. He hardly feels the child; he feels his own emotion and its release. When the slap is given in cold blood, and the adult is not conscious of anger but only of his duty to enforce the law, he may feel even less, and the effect of alienation in the child may be even greater. The comradely slap on the back which friends give each other may sometimes be mutual reassurance and the pleasure of contact, but it may also signify, "Our understanding requires you to accept my superiority and my aggression!"

Our slapping, therefore, no matter how friendly the intention, is apt to have a great deal of unconscious symbolic value and must be studied attentively. In particular, is it our friend's back we are slapping, or his head? If his back, is it the sturdy regions of the shoulder blades or the sensitive area of the kidneys? How can one slap, or tap, the eyes, the lips, the many very different tissues in the vicinity of the ears? Is one conscious where are muscles that need a going over, and where are glands that do not? How deep in the obscure regions between spine and skull, or between spine and pelvis, can slapping bring a new flow of vitality?

In case the reader should already be impelled to try this out for himself, I would suggest he start with tapping his head, where there is a vivid and immediate possibility of exploring and savoring the difference between the delicate tissues enveloping eyes, ears, nose, and jaws, and the solid bone, so close in the neighborhood, where these tissues are attached. Similarly, how deep a stimulation do we need between the lower part of the skull and the back of the neck? But each of us can find out for himself what feels most needed.

Charlotte is convinced that the origin of the practice of spanking children was the primitive impulse to wake them up for things, and not to punish them. However that may be, it is certainly the case in Zen practice, in which a flat, heavy stick is used by the priest to give a resounding and smarting slap to the shoulder muscles of those sitting in meditation who seem in danger of wandering or falling asleep. Sounding in every respect like a severe punishment, this slap is nonetheless regarded by everyone as a helping hand and is often asked for by the recipient, who bows humbly before and after, as does the priest who gives it. To give such a blow effectively, with maximum startlingness and without injury, requires the same kind of knowledge and dedication, with the same amount of practice behind it, as a shot to the green does for a golfer. Such precision is of course not needed for the impact of a hand on a child's buttocks. But in the impulse behind the action, I think every child deeply senses the difference between a spanking administered as punishment for a forbidden act and one given in order to startle him into a larger awareness.

One can approach slapping either as a performance or as improvising and do a very good job in either case. But the way of our work is to feel out improvising: to see the need, feel the ability, and let the result happen. The energy needed is then inspired by the desire for and joy in the activity, in which the actual sensation of what is needed does the guiding. For this to be possible, a certain selflessness is necessary. One slaps easily then, gently or briskly or sharply as the need is felt, with no pursed lips or knitted brows and with breath flowing freely.

In the same way, an African drummer can play hour after hour, his tones and rhythms returning incessantly like the ever-varied waves of the sea, with never the lifeless monotony of a metronome, and without fatigue. Seeing such a drummer, one often sees a man in full meditation, transported and absorbed by the reaction of the drum to his touch and by his own total interaction, through the invitations of the drum, with the responses of the dancers.

Such a scene can be rapturous. All present may be carried along on the living rhythms, which rise and react to the motions of the dancers as the dancers react to them. Every face may glisten with sweat, but no one is tired. Eyes are at rest, breathing joyous; every joint and muscle comes into its own, as each single star does on a clear night. All the drummer does to the drum is slap it. But in his slapping he may glow with such devotion as Buddha does in his enlightenment.

God forbid that we feel our partners as drums and use them either for rhythm or for self-expression! That happens all too often. But we can let ourselves be tuned in for the slapping with eyes at rest and breathing sustaining us, and perhaps at moments become one with the living tissues we are working on.

17 SIMPLE CONTACT

Our classes are of no lasting value unless they inspire the student to continue sensing for himself. As one begins to feel the possibility of life's being an endless exploration, any moment can become a moment of being, full of its own significance. At such moments distractions are not needed, or even interpretations. The present experience is sufficient. Living is its own justification. This is why I have given so much space to the experiments in our classes which we do alone, and which the reader can equally try at home if he has the patience and interest.

Nevertheless, we do not live alone. Every glance, every tone of voice, every letter is a form of contact. Every figure in the supermarket or on the sidewalk is an energy field with which, willy-nilly, we come into some kind of relationship.

People come together, or hold themselves apart, in an infinite variety of ways, complex and simple. All this, one way or another, can be our study. But I should like to start at what seems to me to be the beginning.

Almost from the moment of birth, a baby's life falls into a certain rhythm of action and quiet, of which I suppose the most significant, and certainly the most variable, part is in connection with his mother. In the United States the actual connection may be very slight; in the Mexican countryside it may be constant, with the baby either nursing or resting in his mother's shawl against her breast all day long.

In our competitive culture, the experience of inactive, quiet connection is normally restricted to rare moments of falling or being in love, as when two lovers simply walk holding hands or lean against each other on a park bench. With or without actual touch, such communion occurs more often in youth and in old age than in the "prime" of life. This is a phenomenon very well suited to our study. So I shall begin with the description of a class exploring *simple physical contact.*

We may take a few moments at the start feeling out our standing. To come quietly to ourselves first is really a prerequisite for coming to another. Then we will take partners, preferably someone we don't know and do not choose. One now stands at the side of the other; and when the other signals that he has come to a quiet standing and is ready to be approached, the first person brings his hands somewhere to the other's front and back. Let us say one has come to the other's upper chest and to the back opposite, between the shoulder blades.

What does each feel between the enclosing hands? Time will be needed to come to enough quiet so one can really tell. Does anything change under the touch? If there are signs of life between his hands, does the toucher touch in such a way as not to disturb what he feels living there, yet without diminishing his connection to it?

In actual working, if such questions are asked, long pauses are allowed after each so that everyone has time to let an answer come in its own way. Is it possible to give oneself to sensing without thoughts? Can one feel the difference when now and then thinking is given up—as well as the effort not to think?

After a while we may move. We may come to the lower chest or to the diaphragm; to opposite sides of the head; to the belly, in front and back or at the sides—resting in between and renewing our standing, so that we may be fresh for each experience.

It has been made clear that one partner will bring his hands to the other but *will not manipulate him.* This may not be easy. One may understand that the hands are not to be active: for instance, that we are not to stroke or massage. But simply to come into full, permissive contact with another person is something many of us have been conditioned against since early childhood. We have been taught that we must be in control of ourselves and of our contact with the other—even if only

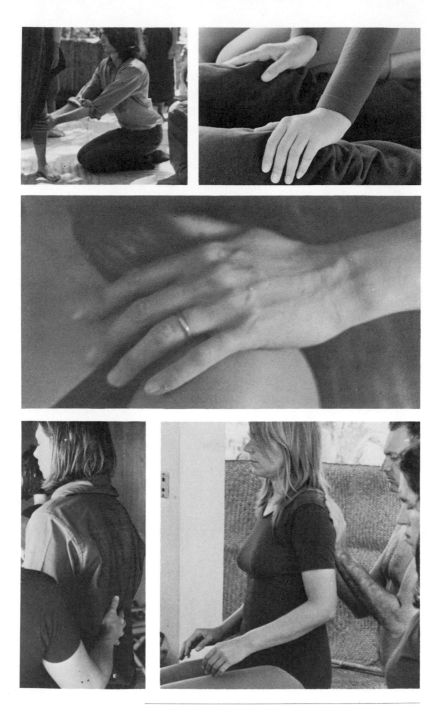

With flexible and quiet hands a dimension enters
consciousness which the eyes alone cannot provide.

through trying to convey the message that we like or dislike him. Unconsciously, we may control our contact and in so doing interfere with our own sensations and direct the other's. Although unconscious, this is already manipulation.

We are actually working when we touch one another—working to try out our hands not as agents of our will but as organs of perception. For this all their native sensitivity and flexibility must be gradually rediscovered.

Even when we have gained freedom to find and adjust ourselves to the structure of the other, it may not be easy to sense and adjust to his balance. If we come to him rigidly, the fine nuances of balance are lost. If we come openly and sensitively, it may help him to a release in which his balance changes, which we must then follow. There is constant change, for this is no mechanical equilibration but the ever-renewed coming into equilibrium of living beings.

Indeed, however we touch him, we may somewhat disturb our partner's freedom. Our hands may feel hard to him, or heavy, or light and fluttery. He may feel "handled," restrained, pressed, or—sometimes a very disappointing experience—not really touched at all. Accordingly, one might expect such contacts to be often unsatisfying, if not downright inhibitive. But in a great majority of cases it is just the opposite. The mere fact that one comes to the other quietly and without overt manipulation is normally very moving to the person touched. He feels cared for and respected. And the one who touches, if he is really present in what he does, is apt to feel something of the wonder of conscious contact with the involuntary, subtle movement of living tissue.

It is probably on the basis of these experiences more than of any others that "sensory awareness" has swept the country in the last few years. A nation of doers, who seldom touch one another without a specific purpose in mind, and whose touch, if not simply careless, is first consciously and then, as it becomes habitual, unconsciously controlled, are asked to come together just to experience. They are not slapping each other's backs to give reassurance or to show approval, not furtively feeling the other to seek reassurance themselves, not trying to correct or relieve the other, or punish or seduce him, or touching symbolically as in kiss and handshake. They have come together only to experience the other, to permit contact in which, even through their clothes, an exchange of vitality occurs simply because we are all alive and give off energy and have the senses and consciousness to perceive aliveness whenever we arrive at the degree of quiet that makes this possible. When even a little of our usual purposiveness is given up, so much aliveness comes through that we are all affected by it.

To permit simple contact is to permit, and necessarily to experience, the natural reinforcement that the living has for the living. It is the experience of mother and infant after breast feeding, when she perhaps rocks him quietly in her arms. It is the shared experience of two survivors of a catastrophe; the experience of peace after a sexual connection that was not maneuvered. It is the experience of just stepping from the inanimate world of the indoors into the living world of a garden. Now, perhaps for the first time, it is asked of one specifically, as simply as one would ask another for a glass of water. No wonder almost everyone is "touched," in fact "moved"; and no wonder we can and do work at this for years, gradually finding a freer opening of those intricate inner passages which inhibit or permit the flow of experience.

It may at any point be helpful, during such experiments, to make time for an interlude of exploring our own hands, or the hands of another, exactly as we explored our feet in an earlier chapter. Though we have not kept our hands packaged all day, as we have our feet, but may have been constantly using them, we have tended to use them over the years in ever more characteristic ways, so that we can often tell one another by our handshakes almost as by our tones of voice. But if our hands are really to find their way to the shapes they come to, they must begin to give up this acquired character and regain their natural potential. For this, a thorough digging into their structure and kneading through of the musculature can be very helpful. The pleasure that attends rediscovery of one's native mobility is a powerful antidote to the habit that is always tending to diminish it. Then, when we come back to seeking the

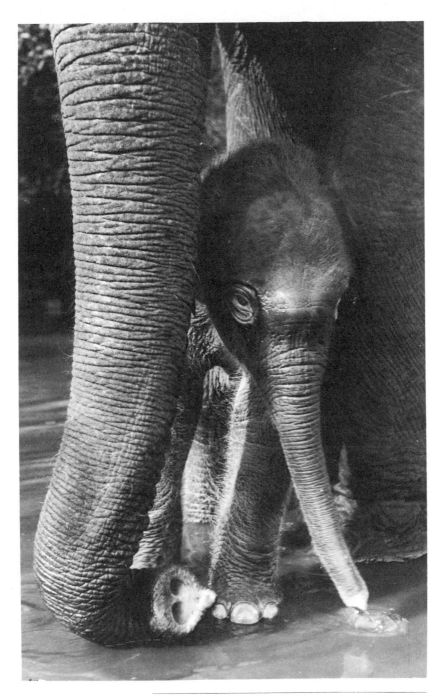

The natural reinforcement that the living
has for the living.

contours of our partner, there is the added interest in feeling our own yielding.

Any number of variations are possible on the basic experiment I have just described. It can be a great joy to let one's hands come fully and feelingly to another's head. So much sensation is latent in the contour of a forehead, or in the complex joining of bone and muscle where neck meets skull. Here, where so many headaches have their seat and so much misery may lodge, is also tissue that rejoices in contact, as every mother knows who has supported the heavy head of her baby or laid a quiet hand on his brow when he had fever. Every owner of a dog or cat knows these spots also, and every lover of a horse. Our habit, of course, is to stroke or scratch or pat, and certainly much of our reward is the animal's active response. But if we would try just coming into contact with the same care and interest that we work toward in the classes, bearing in mind that our pet's sense of time and rhythm is very different from our own, we might find an astonishing new depth of relationship and an unfamiliar equality.

There may be an equal richness in holding another's feet or enclosing his knees. Then one may learn why photography can never replace sculpture. For with flexible and quiet hands a dimension enters consciousness which the eyes alone cannot provide, no matter how deep their gaze or how fine their focus.

Contact may equally be explored when two touch each other: for example, in standing, with each bringing his hands to the hands of the other, or to the other's shoulders. The eyes may be closed, or our gaze may be lowered, so that we see only our partner's form and breathing.[1] Conscious to permit our own breathing, we may compare the way we come to the other with the way we come to the floor, heedful of the question: are such comparisons made with a critical mind and eye, as we have been taught, or just through sensing?

And if the two partners come to movement, is there a movement possible in which neither one leads or urges, where eyes and mind are at rest, where the two become one living bridge

1. Students of Zen may readily see a connection between this attitude of the eyes and their own practice.

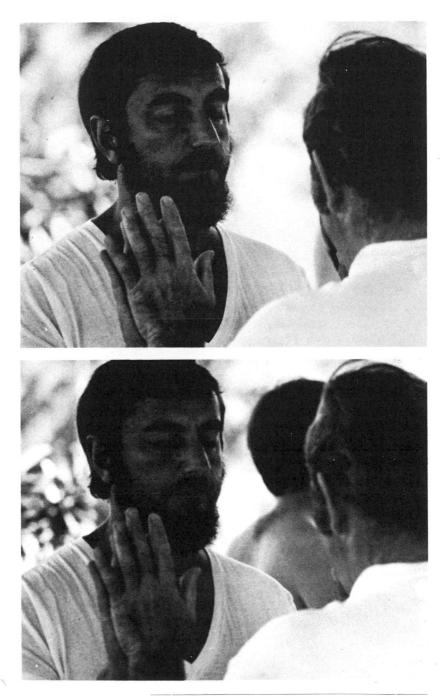

Are such comparisons made with a critical mind
(compare brows) or just through sensing?

from the floor beneath the feet of one to the floor beneath the other?

But do our eyes not meet? Do we avoid this consummation of contact? In any such class as I describe, certain people will find it extremely uncomfortable to forgo looking the other in the eye. In this age of encounter, the reader may well wonder why I suggest deliberately keeping the eyes closed or lowered.

Furthermore, when I suggest a nonvisual or semivisual human connection—especially one that may come into semivoluntary or even involuntary movement—does not so fully sensory a contact lead to the sexual? I feel I should end this chapter with a few words of personal opinion about ocular and genital contact—the two modes which seem to me the most all-pervasive in one sense, and the most highly focused and vivid in another. In these modes, too, the distinction between simple and complex is relevant.

Like our sexuality, I believe the use of our eyes has become compulsive. Impatient with the fears and hesitations implicit in so many of our childhood backgrounds, we seek *breakthroughs* rather than feel our way with quiet and forbearance into more natural organismic paths. In our modern American belief that there is a shortcut to everything, there is a very widespread tendency to try to achieve deeper contact through direct use of the eyes—a sort of cutting of the Gordian knot. It is true that this may have powerful, often immediate, effects. But it is not sensing. To gaze into another's eyes, except in love or in long-tested friendship (when it is sometimes, but rarely, needed as reproach or as reassurance), results in a suspension of sensing, not a deepening of it. To gaze so is more often to declare oneself to another than to perceive him, and to challenge rather than invite the other's response—not to speak of those many occasions when one simply tries to outstare the other. For we Americans seldom have the eyes we had as young children, innocent of competition or intent. We have not the simple fierce, friendly, or evasive eyes of simpler cultures, or the open, inquiring eyes of animals. We can work toward this most natural of all modes of contact, but I do not think we can hurry it. In our classes, when we have gained the courage to feel it is not *evasive* to avoid the other's eyes, we may venture a glimpse of them as we might venture a glimpse of the sun, adjusting the shutter speed of our camera to the energy that can pour instantly through these apertures on a clear day and more slowly on an overcast one. In my feeling, more than that is not generally useful for this study—at least not until very advanced stages of it. "Eyeballing," however useful it may seem as a technique in the field of encounter, calls for a different film from the one we use: an emotional rather than a sensory one. On ours, the result is less likely to be a clear image than plain overexposure.

The eyes were once called the "windows of the soul." When we have worked with ourselves as totalities to the point where we can let our eyes be open to the eyes of another as windows open to the comings and goings of the air, without inhibition to our heartbeat or to our breathing, or to that of the other, then and then only, I should say, can we see with our eyes as true organs of perception and not as instruments of interaction.[2] This, too, we could call "simple contact."[3]

It might seem a similar evasiveness when I say that this work with quiet and reciprocity between partners is neither sexual nor nonsexual. Surely it could be fundamental for love as it could be for friendship, or for dancing, or for a multitude of practical work situations, such as paddling a canoe or moving a piano or setting rafters in a roof—to name a few of which I have experience. But just as we can work over the long haul toward recovery of our innate capacity for a free meeting of the

2. Cf. the extraordinary technique, in Castaneda's books, of scanning a terrain with crossed eyes to perceive differences unnoticeable in normal looking.

3. Our friend Ann Dreyfuss once invited Charlotte and me to the zoo where she worked with disturbed children, encouraging them to come into contact with young animals. It was dusk when she let us in among her animal friends. They showed no signs of fear. Rather, I felt only an intensity and totality of silent presence in the waning light, which in memory I can compare to no other experience. Though the aliveness seemed everywhere, its purest flow seemed to come to me through their alerted heads and especially through their eyes. I have no doubt the actual contact with these animals—even their mere presence—had a therapeutic effect on the children not unlike that which the presence of the Zen master has for his students.

eyes, so our work with simple contact leads ultimately toward an equal and parallel freedom in that other prime facility for relationship, our sexuality.

In a culture where sexuality, like *watching*, has been sharply isolated for the child from the rest of organismic functioning— usually first prohibited and later urgently required—it cannot so easily find its rightful place. But among people who have come to regard orgasm, like a full meeting of the eyes, as something not to be permitted but to be *achieved*, the study of simplicity in contact can be revolutionary.

18 ACTIVE CONTACT

Of course, it is a stirring experience to find oneself yielding with another to a common flow of energy—all the more so when it is not with one person but with several. Who has not thrilled to the sudden, spontaneous wheeling of a flock of birds? In group song or movement—choirs or work gangs chanting, tribes dancing— often irresistible energies may be released, either to be absorbed naturally into the environment, like waves breaking on the shore, or sometimes, if directed by a common need, to work wonders of achievement. In simple contact with another human being, as described in the last chapter, this mutuality may also be discovered, and a similar, if quieter, heightened sense of being may come with it.

But a far commoner life situation is when we are intentionally *doing* something to or for someone else: when our contacts, in other words, are not simple and mutual, but are vehicles through which one person acts and the other is acted upon. This is the specific situation with regard to doctor, nurse, therapist, masseur, et cetera, and patient; counselor and client; teacher and student. Indeed, it is the normal function of most everyday interactions, in the house and out. Above all, we are constantly doing things to and for our children. And all of this, of course, always with the best intentions.

When we reflect on the many cases in which underprivileged children have grown up to be healthier than the "privileged"— namely, when the parents, though unable to provide material goods or avenues to success, have yet simply enjoyed and trusted their children as human beings—we must reconsider and review all our good intentions. Indeed, as we have heard, it is with good intentions that the road to hell is paved—and not only with the intentions that were never realized, but perhaps even more with those that were.

How sensitively and appropriately we act with another person is therefore a vital part of our study. It will be seen presently that this is scarcely different from how we act with things. It is only more complex. In both cases, what we do is functional only to the extent that our perception is unbiased and our reactivity uninhibited. Hank Aaron hitting a ball for a home run and a wide-awake mother gently and surely picking up her baby are functionally the same phenomenon: the full and direct response to a given situation.

In our groups we have many ways of acting upon another, or of setting up situations in which we could call ourselves "helpers." For example, one person may lie on the floor, while another raises and lowers his arm or leg, rather as I have already described a person raising and lowering his own leg. Of course, there are many more possibilities in the present case, for the one lying can accept the help offered, or resist it, or do the work himself, or go through any combination of the three together. The helper may also act in a great variety of ways, very often unconsciously.

In this experiment, the person lying is asked to take time to become quiet and comfortable, and to signal when he feels ready for the other to approach him. This obviates the reflex reactions which might be expected at an abrupt approach. The other, having kneeled or seated himself where he can work easily, then takes the foot and quietly raises the leg a few inches from the floor, sensing its weight. This weight may change perceptibly while the leg is being supported, as the one lying entrusts it more to his helper, or perhaps retracts it; the helper may even see flexings or relaxings in groins and thighs, and changes in breathing. He supports the raised leg, if possible feeling what is going on in and between leg and trunk, perhaps gently moves it a little this way or that, careful not to force it, and then lowers it to the floor. That is the whole experiment, taking perhaps five minutes. Nine times out of ten, the one lying feels eased, lengthened, and more alive in the leg, and

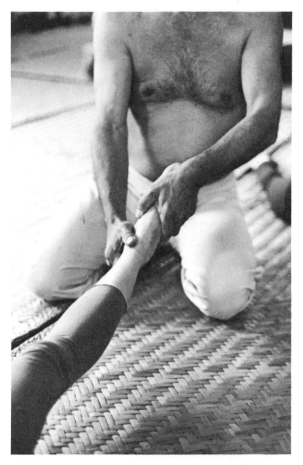

He quietly raises the leg a few inches from the floor.

often throughout the whole side, that was worked with. But what actually happened?

Again, as when we just touched each other, the gratitude at being handled with care by another—at simply not being grossly manipulated—can be overpowering. The mere careful giving of attention is experienced as love. We are still far from any art of loving, as Erich Fromm entitled his book: this is what we shall work at. But in studying this art we shall not be studying techniques, nor shall we be occupied with thoughts of love. For in a garden we do not plant flowers: we bury seeds. If we care for the soil, the flowers will appear by themselves.

When we ask what was experienced, there may well be moving statements about trust and kindness. But we must explore specific details. Was the leg heavy or light? Often it was very light, when one reflects on it, and indeed the helper may recall that the lying one did much of the work himself, instead of letting himself be carried. Was the lying one conscious of this? Usually not. But perhaps there is a memory that the helper did not offer enough security, or seemed unsure, or shifted position while helping, or perhaps gripped too hard, any of which may have made a full entrusting of the weight difficult. Or he may have moved too fast, not giving the one lying enough time to sense the situation fully and to accept and permit the movement offered. So the latter controlled it, either by resisting or by doing it himself.

If so much was imperfect, then, why in so many cases did it move the one helped—now and then to tears? Perhaps because, taking time, the helper sensed what was inappropriate and allowed a change, which caused the one helped to allow change too. And for just a moment a door, which no one knew was there, opened to allow a glimpse into the world of real connection.

Just as the leg may have seemed too light, it may have seemed too heavy. This is almost never because someone is physically unequal to the task. In either case the person lying was probably unable at that moment to allow something to be done to him. Either he guided the activity, or the muscles in his pelvis locked against it. For his part, the helper, meeting the unwillingness to yield, may have been impatient and tried to shake the leg or break through the resistance, thus only increasing it.

Furthermore, a great many people have never really practiced lifting anything, and neither in sitting nor in any other way have adjusted themselves carefully to what the task calls for. Struggling, as a consequence, with what they do, they are unable to offer the calm and security which invites yielding. Finally, a few people will find their leg was pushed unpleasantly into the hip joint, instead of being gently freed there.

Yet, after a few attempts, in which people have had time to get over the novelty of the experiment and come a little more sensitively and discriminatingly to what they are doing, almost everyone will enjoy the experience. When it is really worked with, this can be a very full and beautiful experiment. For with the acceptance, even if only tentative, of another's support, with the beginning of a free yielding to the other, comes the recognition, deep in the tissues, that human contact is not necessarily manipulative, but can be supportive and giving.

I have said that we shall not be studying techniques or seeking a "correct" way to do it. Our study is the soil in which the plant grows. If this soil seems hard, we can find means to loosen it; if we see weeds, we can pluck them. We shall simply work at coming to more quiet and fuller presence in a task, with fewer thoughts and senses more open. In such a task as lifting another's arm or leg, we can see with our eyes and feel with our hands what is asked of us.

Very simply, the question is none other than the title Charlotte once chose for a workshop: *being all there*. Not just

An entirely new connection afterward with the support of the floor.

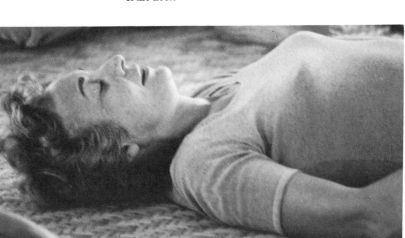

there mentally, as this phrase is often intended, but all there in back, belly, arms, legs, mind, and heart for what one is about to do. When this is true, breathing will be there also.

For instance, many ways of sitting will be inappropriate. They will make a full participation in the task impossible. But as one's interest grows and one finally becomes fully aroused to the task, most people will begin to work from a sitting or kneeling in which the act of raising the leg naturally entails a certain gentle pull away from the trunk, this being a position which also brings all the faculties of the helper into play, including the free flow of his energy and unhampered breathing. The experiment will then be experienced as easy and pleasurable by all concerned; and the one helped will usually feel clearly liberated and in an entirely new connection afterward with the support of the floor.

This last is of the greatest importance, for the sensations of giving and receiving with another person are just part of the larger question of how we give and receive generally in our relationships, and in particular with the ever-present air around us and the support under us. The helper is just a means, albeit a living one who feels and enjoys his part, to awaken us to the whole environment.

19 WORKING WITH OBJECTS

Most of us are interested by the invitation to work with another person. But often we find it difficult to be fully present in the task. Instead of seeing and feeling the one we work with, we are occupied in self-evaluation. Are we doing it right? Are we being sensitive? How do we come across to the other? Do we communicate friendliness, strength, caring, and so on?

All these considerations are barriers between the two, reflecting the attention of the helper back upon himself and diminishing his contact. Equally obstructive is the tendency to apply some technique one has learned for handling others. And a major obstacle is a critical attitude toward the one helped. To recognize our partner's muscular reactions to our offer of help is essential. This is his nonverbal, usually unconscious, communication to us, which speaks directly to our intuition. It is only by such recognition that we can proceed appropriately. But to criticize or evaluate, as we have been trained to do, is to interpose thought formations between ourself and the other, and thus to lose the direct and full connection which is all we have to guide us.

It may be helpful now to begin working with inanimate objects, which cannot preoccupy us so. Any object will do. In fact, the ideal choice would be the things we work with anyhow in daily living: knives and forks, packages, furniture, chinaware, zippers, as well as all professional and playing materials. Charlotte and I find it very convenient and agreeable to work with stones, of which so many beautiful examples may be found on beaches and in river beds all over the world.

What can one learn of a stone? In the first place, it is just there. It has no useful purpose, reveals no intention or direction, and has no interest in us. But it very definitely exists.

If we hold the stone where we can see it clearly, it may have an engrossing form and pattern. But if we close our eyes, all changes: pattern and color are gone; very likely, it suddenly becomes cold. We probably feel something of its form, and we also feel its weight.

How could we feel its weight more clearly? Many people will jiggle and grip the stone, trying to calculate. But are there changes we could allow in ourselves that would let us feel more clearly? For instance, does the wrist let the sensation of the stone through? And the elbow? And the shoulder? Perhaps it involves our way of sitting altogether. Does it involve breathing?

This may become difficult and tiring. Instead of feeling the weight of the stone more clearly, we feel our own difficulties. It is the old problem of being conscious *of* ourselves, not *in* ourselves.

Let us open our eyes and pass the stone to the other hand. To the new hand, it has a fresh form and clearer weight. What do we feel of it now, when we do not look at it? How do we hold it? We may notice now that we are gripping the stone with thumb and fingers, or clutching it, when all we are asked to do is support and feel it. If we relax our grip, we can still feel

What can one learn of a stone?

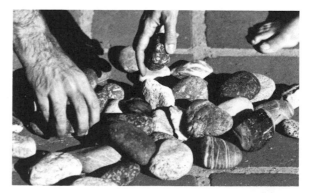

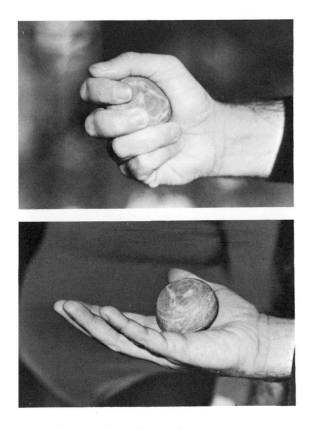

We must neither grip nor lose touch.

its weight on our open palm, and the stone still has the mere
surface it needs under it to be kept from falling.

But now something else has happened. Where is the shape?
We lost it as we relaxed. Yet its shape was just what gave it
individuality.

We realize that to find the stone we must neither grip it
nor in any way lose touch with it. We must feel and give up
our tendency to choose between controlling and withdrawing.
Indeed, the recognition may come, to one who is ripe for it,
that to find the stone we must at the same time find ourselves
—our own flexible, sensitive, inquiring nature. In palms and

fingers, some of us now begin to seek the stone, as perhaps we once sought our own belly, or another's shoulder, coming to it everywhere, without stress, for finer perception.

After a while, we may want to pause and rest. Then we will come to a fresh sitting and take our stone again. Someone remarks that the stone's temperature has meanwhile changed. So a stone is not changeless. Also we find its shape changes as we come to it differently: rounder, if we hold it on one side, flatter if on the other. Let us make an experiment. Let us squeeze the stone. It resists the squeeze. What do we feel of it now, other than its hardness and the pressure we have created on our own tissues?

Let us gradually give up the squeezing until the stone again just rests in our hand. Has anything happened to its weight? Many people will probably report that when they squeezed the stone hard it had virtually no weight at all.

Such experiments can be of prime importance for us. We are immersed in a culture of statistics, standards, and measurements, in which we approach the world only indirectly, as through a Sears Roebuck catalogue. It is not just that it is undoubtedly convenient to buy and sell by the pound, or to take an invalid's temperature. We seek the abstract symbol for its own sake: baseball scores, personality-assessment ratings,

To find the stone, we must at the same time find our own flexible, sensitive, inquiring nature.

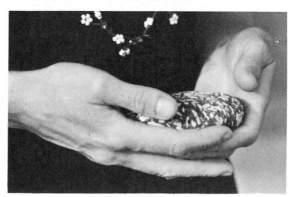

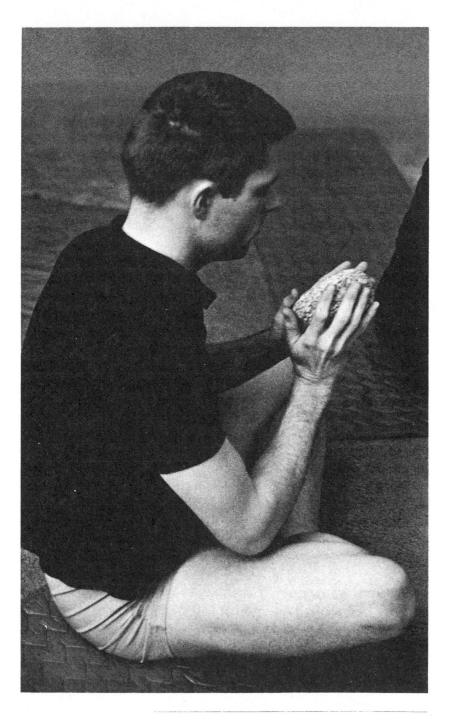

Our sense of its form and weight.

body counts. In the words of General Semantics, we mistake the map for the territory.

In other words, we judge things not with our senses and experience, but by reference to some third, purely conventional factor. Our stone will always bring the pointer of a well-made scale to the same point, which clearly proves the contrary of what we have just discovered: that a stone's weight can change. But as children, our experience was unequivocal that the same snow was at one moment a delight and at another a misery, that the walk to school was short one day and long another, and that a stone which weighed very little when we were feeling well might be heavy indeed when we were sick. And we find that everywhere, just beneath the surface of our conventional "objective" world, lies waiting a forgotten world of overwhelming authenticity, which is not alien but is *ours*.

It has become clear that what we perceived of a stone depended *on how we behaved to it*. When we found our way to a gentler and fuller connection, we perceived more, just as was the case in working with a partner, and just as the floor became softer, or more giving, as we gave more ourselves.[1] Our sense of its form and weight, which tended to disappear when we either acted on it or tried to relax, reappeared as its essential characteristics when we felt out what was needed just to come to it perceptively and in support. When we go now to wash our dishes or our clothes, or to prepare our raw ingredients for cooking, these important tasks—which our culture has labeled as unpleasant and menial, and which industry

1. Cf. page 30. The American man's (and very often the American woman's) fear of *softness*—being a "softie," seeming "soft" on crime, communism, et cetera, with its frequent implications of effeminacy and sexual impotence—is matched only by the assiduousness with which we shun hard furniture; "hard" tasks and chores, for which we seek machines; inclement weather; "hard" facts; and other *hardships* taken for granted in healthier cultures. I am sure this is associated with the profound and very widespread misconception which associates phallic hardness not with the tonicity of the organism but with the hardness of the musculature. The consequent association of softness and yielding with weakness, and of hardness with strength, may account for a great deal of the insensitivity and cruelty of much of our foreign policy, for our anesthetic furniture and automobiles, and for many of the fears and rigidities Charlotte and I are faced with in our classes. It also explains the reactionary rage against "permissiveness."

would deprive us of altogether—may become quite as interesting as driving a car and much more satisfying than television. Truly, when we come awake for what exists in space, there is no need to "kill time."

Some years ago in New York, Charlotte gave a joint seminar with Alan Watts on the Japanese tea ceremony. Alan spoke first in the morning, dwelling on the history of the ceremony and its relation to Zen. Then, for an hour, Charlotte worked with the group on coming to quiet, coming from standing to sitting, and, when sitting, reaching out to touch a stone on the floor. In the afternoon there was a similar division of theory and practice. The second morning, Alan put on his Buddhist robes, set out the hibachi, bowls, dipper, and other paraphernalia of this ancient ritual, and demonstrated the nature and function of each item. Charlotte then worked, as I have just described, on sensing the weight of stones, picking them up and setting them down, and finally giving and receiving stones among the group, bowing to one another meanwhile. By noon, the quiet elation and sense of connection among the different people was very marked. In the final session that afternoon, Alan asked three people to sit in front of the group opposite him, on folded legs, Japanese fashion, while he brought the water to a boil, formally cleaned the bowls, measured with the sliver of bamboo the bright green powdered tea, ladled out the scalding water with the bamboo dipper, whisked the tea into a froth, and, raising each bowl like a sacrament, offered it with a bow to his bowing guests.

Few of the participants had ever seen anything like this outside a cathedral. They were watching in awe. When it was over, there was a quarter-hour interval while people stretched their legs. In the meantime, helpers brought two large bowls of water into the studio, one soapy and one clear, a few dish towels, about thirty plates, and a platter of cookies. The group reassembled. When all were seated, Charlotte asked one person to reach over and take a plate, try its weight, and pass it on. When each could allow his breathing to be at ease for the plate he received, he was to set it before him on the floor. Another person then offered the platter of cookies. Each recipient brought his palms together and bowed in the Japanese *gassho* before taking a cookie, and each held the cookie until all were served. Then all took one bite, tasted, and finally ate. Many reported later that they had never really tasted a cookie before.

Of course the dishes were not soiled, but it was now that the most significant part of the experiment began. The person nearest the bowl of soapy water took his plate there, washed it with a dish cloth, dipped it in the bowl of clear water, and carefully dried it with a towel. All the others watched spellbound. When he had set the dried plate on the floor, folded the dish towel, and come back to sitting, the next one arose.

With thirty people, there was, of course, not time for each to go through the whole procedure alone, so presently a short line had formed by the bowl of soapy water. Charlotte asked if those standing in line were only waiting for their turn, or whether they could become more fully present for the plate in their hands, letting arms and shoulders open for it, letting breathing support it.

There was no need to think. Each could see for himself that whether in the marvelous equipment and ritual of the tea ceremony or in the simple washing and drying of a plain china dish all the elements of sensing and reacting were involved, all the grace and magic of a human presence.

Later, in very different circumstances in Los Angeles, we encountered one man who had never been present at any such seminar. It was in a glorified lunch counter that specialized in steaks and salad. The man was the cook, and his domain was the whole area including the counter where we sat, the adjoining counters where plates were stacked in self-leveling sinks and where great bowls of salad stood, the oven full of baking potatoes, the refrigerator full of a number of different kinds of steaks, and the black grill, framed in gleaming stainless steel, where anywhere from six to a dozen steaks might be cooking at once. In and out slipped waitresses, taking orders which they tucked silently into a revolving rack, and serving the dishes, while two helpers carried new plates in and old ones out, slit and buttered the potatoes, and now and then boldly flung a steak on the grill.

All the men were black, tall and muscular; they might have been either prizefighters or dancers. Some of the waitresses were black, and some were white. But though all were alert and fully occupied, with the ceaseless flow of customers in and out, and had obviously been hired for their speed and efficiency, the whole scene was as though staged for the central figure of the cook, who moved as effortlessly as a brook rippling among the rocks, in every direction, often in several directions at once, with each arm acting on its own as the many details of his job presented themselves, while still in concert with the other.

The whole man stood or moved with the utter equilibrium of a fish in water, and though his movements were as swift as those of a fish, there was no hint of haste or urgency. When one could see his eyes, they were perfectly calm. His lips and cheeks were at ease, his whole form the very image of well-being. No furrow of concern marked his brow, no sign of thought or concentration. But each steak was flipped or removed exactly at its moment, and each laden plate was set on the counter for the waitresses not only without clatter, but without a sound. One could see that each movement of this man was felt and enjoyed through to its very end, while the end of one movement flowed into the beginning of the next with the ease and inevitability of a sleeper's breathing.

For years, each time Charlotte and I were in Los Angeles, we sought out this scene and waited, if possible, for ringside seats. If life is thought of as a dance, I had never seen a more consummate dancer. On the stage, in a setting where he could have been judged by connoisseurs, he might have become a world figure. But in fact he was only a perfectly efficient cook.

One year, when we came back, he had been promoted. It appeared that everyone had felt in him the detachment and presence which he evidently had for people as well as for things, and he had been made manager. He stood, smartly dressed, in the vicinity of the cash register, acknowledging customers; and we could see that his eyes were dulling and his waistline swelling. He still stood with grace, but his tools had been taken from him and the significance of his activity destroyed. To everyone else, it was a sign of success; for us an occasion of mourning. Thenceforth, the steaks lost some of their flavor, and we gradually ceased going there.

This man had related to the many concrete aspects of his job as we work to relate to the stones. He reacted fully and immediately, without thought, to all he saw that concerned him, and he felt everything he touched. He did not *do* the work; he merely responded wholeheartedly to what the situation asked of him. His senses were open, his mind quiet and alert in the background in case of need, and his energies freely responsive.

Seeing this man at work, Charlotte and I were brought deep into the reality of what we aim toward, a state where work in the studio and life outside it would be basically akin.

20 WORKING WITH GRAVITY

If there was one aspect that could have been singled out from the total functioning of the cook I have just described, it might perhaps have been his intimacy with the force of gravity. The attraction of the earth on him and on everything he handled was as perfectly matched to his expenditure of energy as the two lenses of a binocular match when they are brought into focus. Nowhere in his movement was any uncertainty, nowhere an excess. The extension of his arm and the delicacy of his powerful hand when he turned a steak on the grill might have graced the Parthenon; when he set a plate on the counter, the instant when china met formica was exquisitely felt. What made it so stirring to behold was that this perfection was obviously in no sense intended as a performance, but came simply and inevitably from the man's connection with the forces he was dealing with.

It is a misfortune that most of our work must necessarily be done in an empty room. Things come so graphically to people when they can work with their familiar, everyday activities. Once at Esalen Institute we managed to try an unusual experiment. Normally, there was a kind of running battle there between the staff of employees, who tended to feel that Esalen was their private commune, and the "seminarians," who left the square outer world for weekends of what the staff may have often justly regarded as *avant-garde* slumming. In our case, this battle seemed to express itself in a little extra clatter when tables were set in the adjoining room and chairs moved for sweeping.

One day, the kitchen staff was shorthanded, and we were

able to arrange that at a given moment our class would come into the dining room and set all the sixty or eighty chairs on the tables so the staff could sweep. We would then replace the chairs on the floor. It was such an obvious saving for the staff in time and energy that the offer was accepted. The class had been working with stones, and when the moment came it was simple and natural to go from stones to chairs. Each of us took a moment to come into touch with the weight of the chair and to find a good connection with the floor, so we could let it help us. Though any mention of noise or quiet had been carefully avoided, it was almost without a sound that the chairs rose and landed on the tables. Of course, a number of the kitchen staff had come out to watch how the square seminarians would fare with a real-life task, and what they saw surprised them. Pensively, the sweepers swept, and we were called in again. Again the same. As if by their own impulse, the chairs in our hands left the tables and came softly and surely to their places on the floor. We would all have been hired on the spot; and for a day or two the war between the groups noticeably abated.

I wish it might have been practical to do the sweeping too, and gradually to work our way into all the activities being carried on in our neighborhood in dining room and kitchen. In the complexity of Esalen, and the brevity of our stay, such an invasion would of course have been quite impossible. But in the Zen monastery at Tassajara, California, where we work for a week each spring, a few of our students do find their way into every work activity, mingling as harmoniously with the Zen students and monks as the different rivulets that mingle in Tassajara creek. What in most cases would be felt as an intrusion into kitchen, shop, and cupboard here becomes a natural union. So people work when the work is noncompetitive, based only on a common perception of need and sense of capacity. Elsa Gindler, the originator of our studies, often worked with her students on sweeping and mopping the floor, relating the energy mobilized to the work to be accomplished.

But we can work with our stones. Gravity has no preferences. The same forces and elements are involved. So if we sit again and take a stone, we can come to a new start.

As we hold the stone in our hand, sensing its shape and weight, we may quietly feel first what changes might need to be allowed in our sitting for more inner freedom and easier breathing. This may also bring about changes in the weight of the stone. What *is* the weight? Not how much, but *what*? As it begins to occupy our attention, it may occur to us that the weight of our stone is merely its tendency to lead us somewhere, stronger in one stone and weaker in another. Where would it lead us, if we should follow it? To follow, of course, would mean not to interfere with it. We make the attempt: it is not so easy not to interfere. We have too many knees and elbows, too much of our own weight to contend with: perhaps there is just too much of us altogether.

To find out what is happening, we may ask someone to sit in the middle and work alone, letting the stone follow its weight to the floor while the others watch. The stone descends irregularly. Another person tries. This time the stone clearly goes down on a slant.

What is the problem? We study the experimenter's behavior. Is he with the experiment? Not altogether. For one thing, he is frowning. That means that something is busy controlling something else, not following the stone. Also, his shoulder may be cramped, as though pressing something under his arm which isn't there. He seems somehow uncomfortable in sitting and perhaps distracted by this from the slight changes needed as the stone sinks. Or perhaps he is judging its course downward with his eyes, as though he could see where weight *should* lead, thus dividing and distracting his attention from where it *does* lead.

We realize that it would be a miracle if anyone were so flexible and so reactive throughout that he could fully allow the stone to lead him.

Then why work at it, if it is an impossible task? . . . But let us try once more.

We sit, holding our stone, eyes closed. Where does it lead?

Now the leader may ask, "Are your eyes quiet?"

No, they are not. Behind our closed eyelids, we can feel the effort to see what is going on.

Or he asks, "Do you allow breathing?"

As each question sinks slowly into us, something does awaken inside us and perhaps seeks unforeseeable new adjustments. We seem to open inwardly for the stone. It becomes more present to us; we can sense where it would lead us and begin to follow it. That is not all. Having given up something we cherished, some of our control, we have also become more alive. This has happened because we have begun to give ourselves to a task. Perhaps to fulfill the task is not so important as just to give ourselves to it, whether it seems impossible or not.

To a casual onlooker, the slight inner changes might be unnoticeable. But to one who could see—even though the stones may still slant and falter—each of us might now radiate an aura of quiet and presence.

We can take another approach: we can have the stone on our head.

In preparation, we come to standing. Standing has something to do with letting our weight go down to the ground. If we feel that in some way we interfere with this, we take time to sense through and give up what we can of the interference. Changes in balance may follow, more granting of freedom in neck or back, more elasticity in ankles and feet, and so on.

If we now place the stone on our head, could this slight additional weight also be allowed consciously down through us to the ground? Whether we hold it up or not, the ground receives it anyhow. It is only we who come into strain when we resist the passage. Obviously, we can no longer grip the stone, as we could when we held it in our hand. But someone may now feel that his neck is gripping his head, so as not to let the stone fall off. Or that he is holding his breath, or in some other way behaving apprehensively. If we become conscious of anything like this and find that we can give it up, there is a sensation of relief and many changes may occur simultaneously.

Of course, if we just try to "relax," we will lose not only unneeded tensions, but needed ones also; in short, we will lose touch with floor and stone. Unless the stone is quite flat, it will probably fall—a happy consequence, since it may startle us awake. But if we give up only what interferes with sensing our way into fuller connection with stone and floor, this will lead us to a more balanced standing and into a clearer relationship with the whole environment, including ourselves, in which we are not so much holding the stone up as merely permitting ourselves to rise under it, as we rise naturally in our reaction to gravity.

Our weight, plus that of the stone, is allowed down to what easily and surely receives it beneath us; our full natural stature is allowed up. On top of all rests the stone. Beneath lies the earth.

21 DOWN AND UP

What is it that we have discovered so far in working with our stone? Among other things, the stone had temperature, form, and weight, each of which properties was perceived according to our own condition. To each of these aspects of its existence we have corresponding modes of sensing, and the joints and muscles needed to bring us where our sensing is effective.

We have been working mainly with weight, and we found that when our attitude to the stone changed, the sensation of its weight changed correspondingly. But this was not true of the direction in which its weight led us. Whether the course we followed seemed irregular or slanted to those who watched us, to us it always seemed *down*. If our sense of direction does not agree with that of others, there must somewhere be an impairment of perception. For if we let the stone drop, it is clear to everyone, including ourselves, that it falls in one direction only. Our impairment is evidently not visual, or in our sense of verticality, but must be in our kinesthetic sense, or ability to feel our own muscular activity and simply give to the weight of the stone. We are not sensitive enough to be able to tell just when we are yielding to gravity, and when we are exerting another force of our own.

Anything so ever-present as this pull of gravity, which leads the stone always to fall in the same direction, must be worth our study. I should more properly call it the pull of the earth, for that is all that concerns our personal experience. In its subtle ways, this pull is at work on us all the time. Furthermore, with a little reflection, we may realize that the direction of this pull, in which the stone falls, and in which, with more or less

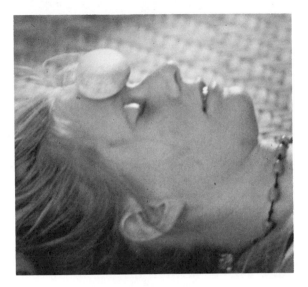

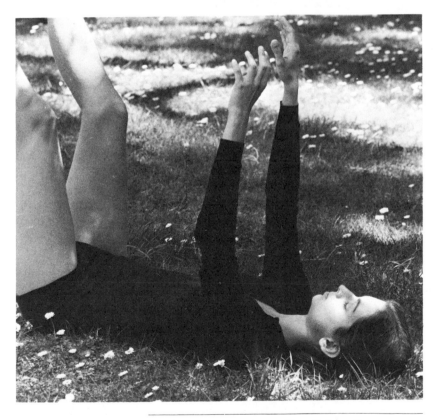

Anything so ever-present as this pull of gravity.

clarity, we can feel ourselves being drawn also, differs in this respect of constancy from all other directions whatsoever. Day or night, fog or sunshine, it is always there, independent of compass, or rising and setting sun, or north star. It is unrelated to any of our five senses at all and is perceptible to us only through that all-pervasive inner reactivity, the proprioceptive or kinesthetic senses, without which we could not stand erect or relate to anything around us. When we take time to come to more quiet and awakeness, these senses begin to come to life within us everywhere.

We can be sure that every child and every animal reacts instinctively to the pull of the earth; we see that plants respond to a balance between the pull of the earth and the source of light. The direction of this pull is unequivocal. Indeed, it is the only direction in which there has always been something there for us to come to—something, in fact, that with sensitive adjustment we could come to rest on. Perhaps this is one of the reasons why the earth has been called mother, and why something in me, at least, yearns to return to her. This basic direction, *down*, which always is ultimately *down to earth*, is where the stone would lead us, surely and truly, if we yielded to it.

But in working with the stone on our head, we have also discovered something else. When we began to ,approach the flexibility and balance needed simply to allow the weight of the stone down through us to the ground, we at the same time, of necessity, began to allow our own stature up.[1] The inner passages that opened in response to the pull of the earth upon the stone opened also for the flow of energy needed to maintain the height and breadth and depth in us that our organs and tissues require for free functioning. Against our own acquired tendencies to control and constrict, we were obliged to yield upward and outward to our inner needs at the moment when we

1. Cf. "Finding Our Stature," page 54.

Knowing down, we know up.

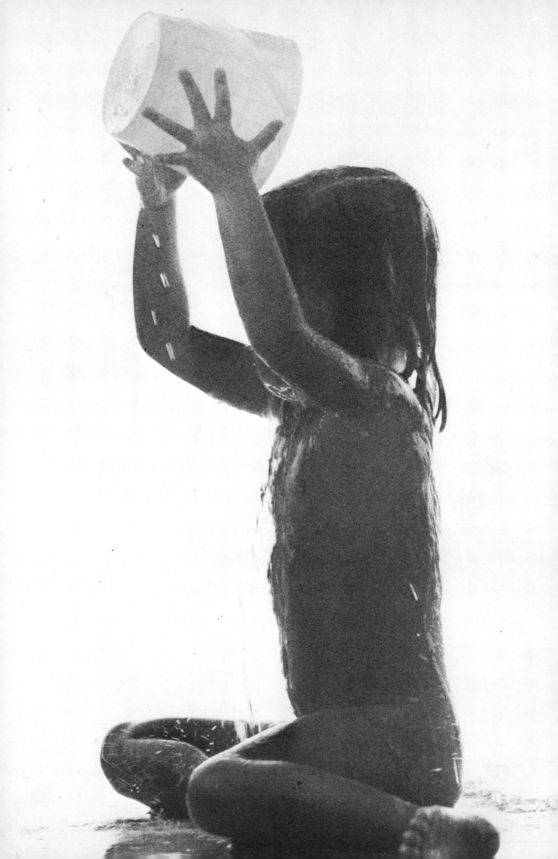

yielded downward to gravity. In this, we were no different from any healthy flower or any blade of grass.

Equilibrium, for human beings as for all other terrestrial creatures, is thus not just a lateral balancing, as of weighted scales, but involves an equally critical balancing of two forces in the vertical, a process which is entirely spontaneous when not impeded by illness or conditioning. What we must yield to, when we are borne upward involuntarily against the pull of the earth, is the spontaneous generation of energy in our own organism. Much of the working of this *metabolism*, as it is called, can be felt. It is what gives the sensation of lightness and well-being. Unless we are sick, the energy needed for standing is supplied automatically; we have only to sense and give up the efforts and constrictions that impede the natural circulation of this energy through arteries and veins. We stand as all animals stand, even elephants, with our full weight, yet freely and effortlessly, and to our full stature, yet with no straining upward. When we tell a child to stand up straight, or to stand taller, as in so many cases we were told ourselves, we are trying to impose voluntary processes upon the fully sufficient involuntary processes given us by nature. This is gilding the lily. Those of us with a military or "aristocratic" bearing, should they practice yielding, would lose none of their stature. All they would lose is their subservience to an image and their isolation from the world of actuality.

In standing, with or without a stone, all that is important is the sense of how our native energies can be allowed free circulation, and of the direction to which they must respond. With this, the stone on our head can be of help to us. As we become quiet and present for it, we feel its weight constantly pressing down through us, eliciting an equal and opposite energy of our own, bringing our limbs and inner masses into a natural alignment toward the earth, which at the same time pulls us toward itself and supports us against its own pull.

Knowing *down*, we know *up*. Knowing up, we freely stand: not otherwise. Sensing and allowing what is needed, we begin again to experience our deep inner capacity to relate to the world.

22 WORKING OUT OF DOORS

The best place to study gravity is not in our classes but in daily life: climbing or descending stairs, carrying bundles, setting the table, serving and washing dishes, getting up and sitting down, dancing, or, perhaps best of all, walking on uneven ground. Our summer students in Maine have often learned more from the rough, woodsy paths and rocky headlands than from anything we could offer them in our studio. Indeed, our chief contribution has been to get them there and then induce them by one means or another to give up both "practical" concerns and daydreaming, and to allow the immediate present to occupy them. In this, we are powerfully aided by the vivid presence of nature.

In walking, one's concern is with the way; but this does not mean being on the lookout for stones and roots, even though that may be prudent and helpful to start with. By and by, we are no longer caught in the opposites of absentmindedness and vigilance. If I "kept my eye on the road," as I drive down Seventh Avenue in New York, it would be as fatal as if I drifted off. In New York traffic, I have had to learn to be open and alert for everything, still or moving, on all sides and behind me as well. I don't look: I only try to be all there.

It is the same walking through the woods or over the rocks. We no more need to "look where we are going" than does a deer or a goat. We have the same faculties as they; we may only lack practice. When we are alert, we see what we need to see and do not stumble. In the same way, we need not struggle up the slopes or hesitate down them. We may want to go a little faster or slower here and there; we may leap down the rocks and come back up them using hands and feet; but as we see the terrain our balance and our energy adjust to it automatically.

We take this for granted in skiing. Without the instantaneous readjustments in balance and energy to the swiftly changing slope, no skier could ever get down a mountain. Skiing, I suppose, is the best of all possible sports for studying sensory awareness. But we are all skiers, in one sense or another, when we allow ourselves to be and take the time for it. The gentler our eyes and the smoother our brow, the more lightly and easily we get there.

Now and then, on the Maine seacoast, we give a whole class out of doors. The group meets in front of the little hotel, and, when we are assembled, we may set out for the great spruce-covered bluff called Burnt Head. It is agreed we will walk the whole way there and back in silence.

As we take the dirt road up the hill, perhaps thirty people altogether, I become conscious of my legs, like those of the horses I have ridden, coming powerfully into action. The others, climbing silently on all sides, make it seem like a cavalcade or a pilgrimage. But these associations are fleeting, soon lost in the complex sensation of the changing terrain underfoot, and of the varying energies I and the others mobilize as it becomes now steeper and now easier. I feel breathing become stronger as I climb; I sense it in the others. In the absence of talk, it is easy to allow less effort, more economy. Walking becomes an experiment in sensing.

The road leaves the houses and shrinks to a trail on entering the woods. Many of us remove our shoes. There are changes underfoot: grass, damp earth, spruce needles, roots, stones. Freed of shoes, we are conscious of each new surface we encounter. Here and there, someone pauses momentarily, testing the dampness or savoring the refreshing coolness of the ground. There are changes in acoustics and temperature too. Among the thickly growing trees, there is not simply an absence of sound. Quiet has a living immanence. One is conscious of a multitude of organisms: trees, undergrowth, plants, grasses. One can almost feel them growing; one can feel their silence and presence. We can feel our own silence as we walk:

each of us with a new dignity when he just exists, breathing, his heart beating, walking with care for the path.

One after another, we emerge from sheltering woods to granite ledges high above the ocean. Among them, exposed to every weather, stand small, pointed spruces. In hollows and crevices, grasses and bayberries grow. There are tiny meadows, with wild roses and daisies among the grass. Everywhere, some hundred feet below, is the vast ocean, a glittering surface wrinkled into endless waves, endlessly approaching, each one at last blossoming in explosions of white foam along the rocks. As the foam recedes, dark seaweed marks the tidelines. Above and beneath us, gulls soar against the blue of the sky, or the darker blue of the sea and gray of the cliffs. The air is in movement on these rocks, and the sea sounds. At so slight a distance, it is another world from the woods we have left.

We have come silently, each one for himself, to some vantage point for sitting or standing, or perhaps for stretching out on the sunwarmed rocks. No one speaks. It is not just our agreement: we are filled with the power of the scene.

And yet soon, in spite of the quiet, and even awe, before nature that has been apparent in the group, cracks begin to appear. Some people are already plainly being lulled to sleep by sun and wind. Others have lost their connection and are now wondering, "What next?" For many, perhaps, the scene begins to shift in and out of reality, becoming more and more a picture postcard, the stereotype of conventional "beauty" and "inspiration"—no longer one's own experience. Here and there, an old cigarette butt, browned by weather, testifies that for others too this place may have been too strong to take pure.

What way is there of coming back to ourselves, of finding a common ground? The question answers itself: *our common ground*. What could be more fitting, after this flood of sensations from without, than to ask everyone to close his eyes, wherever he may be, and feel his way up to standing on whatever is under him, whether bare rock or living vegetation?

The request brings us back into a sense of interaction. We are not merely passive. For some, it may be necessary to survey the terrain first; for others it is secure just as they are. One element all share in common: the absence of any man-made floor.

Wherever we are, the earth's surface is uneven: we must find individual adjustments for each foot and leg, and corresponding adjustments throughout ourselves altogether, coming gradually to an unequal standing that might yet be effortless. Our bare feet, practiced in classes, are now awake to find the shape of rocks and grasses to which we can give our weight, finding contact and using the support for standing freely.

With the visual shut out, we may become very conscious of the feel of the wind and the sound of the surf below. We experiment with covering our ears. Muffling the sounds outside,

Awake to find the shape of rocks and grasses.

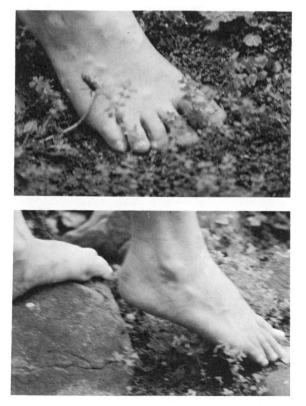

we are overrun with our own interior murmurs. After a time, we remove our hands from our ears. The roar of the sea fills us. Even the earth under us hardly seems as powerful. We allow our eyelids to open. Equal vastnesses of sky and sea spread out before us. Our feet seek assurance in the support beneath. It is no postcard any more.

With open eyes, we may turn slowly where we stand, taking time to feel each new surface as we come to it and to allow a sensitive meeting. The panorama changes as we turn. Everywhere are other living organisms, some like ourselves, turning and finding new adjustments to gravity, others straight as candles in a candelabra—the little spruces, with their outspread rings of branches and tips shooting skyward. The wind moves through the spruces, engendering a multitude of slight movements in their twigs, from which they return ceaselessly to rest. We, too, may be aware of our unceasing inner response to the presence of the air, the delicate commotion of inhalation, and in exhalation the momentary but unfailing pause, also for rest.

It is time to communicate in words. We sit in a close group, while a few verbalize the experiences they wish to share. Then perhaps we all lie down on the many variations of surface which the earth offers.

Though it may be unawares, we have been studying modes of perception. Starting in a situation where sensory impressions are too multitudinous to absorb, we limit ourselves to specific avenues, as one might with a camera. The *gestalten*[1] form and dissolve, each in its given time taking the stage and withdrawing: now we feel the support of the earth and our adjustments to it; now the world comes to us through the threshold of our ears; now it enters through our eyes. Even in the exchange of our experiences we are being focused, this time by words and voices.

Someone has just stated, "I could feel the earth receiving my weight, and myself receiving the air."

1. Organized *phenomena*, the study of which is the field of Gestalt psychology, and whose dynamic, together with much of sensory awareness, underlies Gestalt therapy.

It is not his usual tone of voice: he speaks with a directness and simplicity that draw us to look at him. This is a statement that could easily sound pompous or fanciful, but in his expression is the same genuineness as in his voice. It is as though the experience itself is speaking through him, to which his ordinary mannerisms have yielded. We believe him. Deep in us, something responds. He has brought us again, for a moment, into consciousness of that greater world from which, though we seldom realize it, we are inseparable.

23 WORKING OUT OF DOORS, CONTINUED

In these inviting circumstances, one may work with many variations of our work indoors. But there would be no sense in ignoring the surroundings for which we came here. So we stay with what is specifically offered. The terrain is irregular: we may take hands in a ring and with eyes closed circle over it to right or left, alert not to trip or stub a toe, awake for the hands and the balance of both of our partners, steadying and being steadied without stress or exaggeration. Now, as so often, is a fine occasion for sensing breathing and allowing it free play. Or we may all walk at random over rocks and slopes, feeling through and through the common courtesy of occasionally giving one another a helping hand when it is steep or slippery. Or we may move up and down the slopes on all fours, sensing the redistributions of weight and energy when it may actually be helpful to use hands as well as feet.

We may practice over and over with seeing, closing our eyes and allowing more restfulness in the space between them, giving time for the eyelids to come to resting too, and then letting them open quietly, without looking, to admit the leaves and grasses of the foreground, or the waves churning far below against the rocks, or the horizon between sea and sky. We might borrow from formal studies of meditation and spend five or ten minutes looking only at a single object—a twig or flower, perhaps—following the metamorphoses that occur when our thoughts become quiet and we let ourselves be led into its strange world.[1]

1. I am indebted for this nonchemical psychedelic experiment to Claudio Naranjo, who used it in a joint seminar we once gave together.

Many will be delighted if we avail ourselves of another possibility in our surroundings and pick sprigs of spruce needles and bayberry leaves, crushing them in our fingers to release their fragrance and smelling them ourselves or offering them to others. This too, for all its deliciousness, is an inquiry into our nature and our upbringing. For example, do we sniff actively, as we have seen everyone do when he judges something, and as we have seen animals do constantly, or do we just let it come to us?

What would happen if we didn't sniff? We renew our offerings to find out. The aroma comes to us on quiet inhalation, all by itself, as surely as that of a pie baking in the oven. We have only to be present and awake for it. For comparison, we actively sniff again. Indeed, we smell the fragrance this way too. But there is a difference. In sniffing, the scent is somehow restricted to our nostrils, where it is judged. Our eyes are not at rest; breathing is controlled. Once again, we just let the scent come

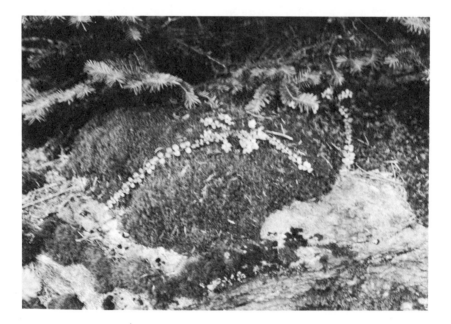

to us. It comes slower, perhaps more faintly, but it pervades us. Something of the essence of tree and shrub mingles with us. We begin to find that even in smelling we have the choice of being either open to the world or manipulative.

As with food at a picnic, almost everything is enhanced in the presence of the fresh air and vegetation, the rocks, flowers, sea, and the lonely, swiftly passing gulls. This is no achievement of ours. It is a free gift. But it can only be given if we are freely there to receive it—which we cannot be if we are occupied in trying to capture it.

When the group was asked to make written reports on one such class, a member wrote, "I am enjoying myself thoroughly. But asking me to report my experience is like asking me to give you a cup of that surf we saw yesterday foaming on the rocks!" Coming from a very articulate landscapist and architect, this was certainly the keenest report of them all.

It so happens that at Burnt Head, besides the rocky ledges and the woods behind them, there is also a little meadow, of perhaps a quarter of an acre, of grasses, wild flowers, and bayberry shrubs. Into this a path leads and disappears. After an hour on the ledges, we may pass through the trees into the meadow for another taste of nature.

Here, wherever we stand, sit, or lie, it cannot but be in a certain sense an act of violence. Not only is this no wooden floor, or bare rock or earth; it is not even a lawn of trimmed and resilient grass, or a pasture grazed by animals which has grown up underfoot. Here the earth is already fully occupied with living things, striving upward in the light and air; we have no choice but to superimpose ourselves upon a scene that was already complete without us.

As we leave the little path and spread out in the meadow, some of us may again be occupied with thoughts and be "absent-minded" to one degree or another. Under these wanderers, the grasses are crushed heavily. But others, whose senses have remained alert, now step fully present into the sun-dappled leafage and quiet of the meadow. For them, a new lightness stirs in blood and limbs, and, for all their weight, they step with a gentler tread. The vegetation is still pressed to earth, but after these more buoyant steps it recuperates faster. One might say these plants have been injured but not insulted.[1]

As we assemble, and each finds a place to stand, the present tends to come into focus for us all. Something of the life process of the myriad living things environing us, some sense of their interaction with earth, air, and light, steals into our blood stream; some of their chemistry intermingles with ours.

Here and there, someone becomes aware of a new subtlety in breathing, or feels an intimation of the exchange between the air and the pores of his skin. Perhaps we are all now asked to close our eyes and sense breathing. In the growing sense of coexistence with nature, we may notice strange inner readjustments. In someone's pelvis, perhaps, or in neck or shoulder

1. Since this writing, publication of *The Secret Life of Plants* by Peter Tompkins and Christopher Bird (New York: Harper & Row, 1973) makes this statement sound quite realistic.

With bare hands, as with our bare feet on the meadow, we come sensitively, in seeking and accommodation, not with intention.

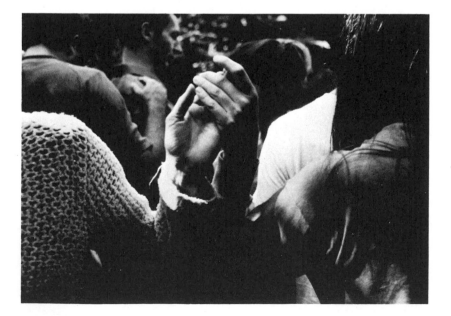

girdle, an old knot may loosen slightly; standing shifts; the ice of some old anxiety thaws a little, releasing rivulets of energy that bring moisture to the eyes or streamings of sensitivity to the soles of the feet. One feels impulses of love for life and for living things.

When we open our eyes now, the meadow may seem radiant in its stillness. If we walk a little here and there, we step with a new sensitiveness and respect, in more conscious connection with the air and with our own weight, and more aware as we come into contact with what we step on.

It may be that two people will come together now, the hands of each coming somewhere to the other. Here too is life. With bare hands, as with our bare feet on the meadow, we come sensitively, in seeking and accommodation, not with intention. Our eyes are not probing, but quiet. Our pores are open. Our energies flow back and forth, as gentle and permeating as the air flowing through our nostrils. Life needs our conscious permission to function freely, and we are practicing permissiveness.

No one finds it difficult to keep our pact of silence when the group finally dissolves into its constituent individuals, who remain meditating where they are, or go off among the trees to the rocks or to the village.

24 THE WORD AND THE VOICE

In the last chapters, I mentioned two reports by students of their experiences. The first, in the simplest words, reported the sensation of receiving the air and being received by the earth. The second, in writing, stated that the experience could no more be verbalized than one could capture the foaming of sea water in a cup. Both were genuine and direct communications; and in the one that was spoken, the speaker's words could be substantiated by his tone of voice. As a rule, most of us spend our lives avoiding both of these alternatives. We neither remain silent in the presence of something really inexpressible in words, as children do, nor do we simply let the experience find its words. This is why the sound of our voice, as well as the facial expressions that accompany it, tends to come from every level of us except our depth.

An infant's expressions, however swift to change, are perfectly unambiguous. No arch smile, or brows knit in concern, stand between what he feels and what we see. No meaningful laugh or sarcastic tones interpret his feelings to our ears. He speaks directly. Yes is yes, and no is no.

But this state of affairs is not normally of long duration. Unlike the instinctual vocal communications of infancy such as screaming or cooing, which convey feelings, speech, consisting of the discrete conventional sounds which we call words, is entirely imitative. But as we learn to imitate the words we hear, and the combinations of words, we unconsciously imitate at the same time the modulations, tones of voice, and variations in emphasis that represent individual or cultural attitudes behind the words. This, of course, is the reason one person's accent can raise the hackles on another's neck. It is also one reason why our words so seldom correspond with our own deep feelings. Yet speaking was, I suppose, the first uniquely human mode of communication, is still of unique importance, and involves a variety of useful nonverbal components far outranging anything available to animals.

It is possible to work on this question. Once, when I was studying in Switzerland with Elsa Gindler's colleague, Heinrich Jacoby,[1] the group spent the entire three-hour morning session on speaking out a single sentence. Jacoby began by asking someone to make a statement; and after a number of unsatisfactory attempts, it being a brilliant day with the Alps snowy white in the distance, someone said, "On such a clear day, one can see the mountains."

We worked the whole morning on sensing what each of us was nonverbally adding to or subtracting from this statement when we tried to repeat it. Each of us could begin to hear when it rang more or less true in the others. Gradually, when it was our turn, we began to feel what was happening inside ourselves.

Of course, any gesture or statement is apt to feel less natural when it seems one is on stage. How, before others, can I repeat an observation as though it had really come from me, spontaneously, then and there? Indeed, if the reader tries it out alone it will probably still seem to be before an audience.

But we were not trying to achieve spontaneity. We were just repeating a simple statement, whose validity each one of us could verify for himself, and trying to become conscious of what actually happened in us when we did so. What did happen was not simply the effect of self-consciousness before a group; it was each one's particular self-consciousness, expressing itself a little differently from everybody else's. In fact, it was what happened anyhow in our normal speaking, only exaggerated in certain ways. The constraint and embarrassment which these exaggerations represented could, of course, easily be felt, but the form their expression took, though easy to perceive in others when one really became interested, was very

1. See Appendix A.

hard to recognize in oneself. We have heard our own mannerisms so often that they have become all but unconscious.

The study of one's own voice can be vividly enhanced by
using a tape recorder. I still recall an experience from the summer of 1948, when wire recorders were just beginning to be
used. My first wife and I, together with my parents, had been
invited for dinner with my brother and sister-in-law. The six
of us sat there talking merrily while, known only to our hosts, a
wire recorder was at work under the table. After dinner, at a
pause in the conversation, my brother announced what he had
done and asked if we would like to hear the results.

There was not much high fidelity in those days, but no one
failed to recognize everybody else's voice in all its normal tones
and mannerisms. Only his own voice, to each one of us, came
as a shock. And what we had supposed was a civilized conversation sounded like a battlefield. It was as though no one
let anyone else finish, but charged in helter-skelter as soon as
he thought he could be heard.

My father turned pale. My stepmother, whose voice was
also "cultivated," listened in amazement and disbelief. For my
part, I was overwhelmed. Traits I disliked in the modulations
of my father's and brother's voices came across even stronger
in my own. Only my brother and his wife, who knew what was
coming, were delighted. Except for them, none of us had ever
before heard his own voice coming to him through the same
channels as the voices of others.

Many readers will recognize here an effective form of therapy which has lately come into widespread use: self-confronta-
tion through the use of videotape. But audiotape alone can provide great revelations. Our voices, unconsciously imitative, are
unnatural. We are used to them, and so is everybody else; they
have become "second nature." But on a tape, we hear them not
only from the outside rather than, as usually, from the inside,
but also removed from the context and situation which occupied our attention as we were speaking. So our own voice comes
to us objectively, so to speak, and we are for once able to hear
not only our words but also all the unconscious overtones
accompanying them, all the mannerisms we have built up to

get by in our particular milieu. Since this is only another way to speak of our conditioning, such a study leads us directly into our basic social attitudes.

Speech is only a special mode of making sound, and in our classes we can work with "sounding" just as can any teacher of voice or singing. But as always, we proceed in the opposite of the usual manner, feeling out what happens and disregarding all accepted standards. We may practice just allowing exhalation to carry sound—*ah, oh, ohm*, or whatever—perhaps feeling with our hands wherever the spontaneously arising vibrations can be felt in us. Or we may bring our hands to another to feel the vibrations in him. It is surprising to find the great range of vibrations possible in one's own vocal cords and the extent of the tissues in us that resound to them. Natural harmonies form readily when such sounding is practiced in a group, even when it is agreed that no one will fall into his familiar patterns. From here to voicing sound is a very natural step: again with the agreement that, with no attempt to be original or different, we will nevertheless strictly avoid the familiar and known, and stay with exploration.

It is only one more step from vocalizing to verbalizing. Word sounds may now be felt, perhaps for the first time, as not only conventional but also organismic expression, in the same way as sounding and singing. Each person has his own individuality. For each, there is a timbre in the sound of words which is natural to his own individual jaws, larynx, shoulder girdle, diaphragm, belly, to his real feelings and interests—in short, to himself. We have always known something a little like this. We can tell our friends more clearly by their voices than by almost any other mode of expression. One may recognize a voice on the telephone that one has not heard for years. But what we have not known is that each of us has another voice, equally ours—indeed, far more deeply ours—that appears once in a great while, like some rare but inconspicuous flower, at certain moments. Such moments may be forgotten immediately, or they may linger in memory with the unaccountable persistence of some trifling dream fragment. But these are the moments when we have spoken spontaneously, not from the eruption of inner pressures, but from the same sense of simple contact that we were exploring in touch. This is when all need to conform has momentarily slipped from us, and we have been simply ourselves.

Just as we may work for years to recover and re-establish the capacity for simple contact, so we may work to find our own voice. With the voice it is more difficult, for we are used to using it constantly, in every kind of situation; while consciously touching another is already something rather special. The first step is simply to begin to hear our own speech.

In a class, one may once in a while call the roll at the beginning, and later, after working, call it again, noticing what are often striking differences in the quality of response. Or, standing in a circle, perhaps hand in hand, or arms over each other's shoulders, one after another may speak out his own name—in many cases a name he does not fully accept. As reinforcement, when one speaks his name, the others may repeat it, each one letting the name be more fully and simply allowed as sound. We might work at this until everyone has said his name several times—not because it is his "turn," but just because he feels the need to try it. This can be very helpful. It is not always easy to say one's name clearly and simply. And few indeed can speak their name to a group without a touch of defiance or, more likely, humorous deprecation. In courtlier times, the act was made easier by adding an "at your service," as is still true in Latin countries today. But when this basic hurdle is over, all other statements become a little easier to make.

25 TASTING

One Easter week, in the early years of Esalen, Charlotte and I were giving a workshop. Mild spring air, bearing a faint scent of ocean and of aromatic shrubs, flowed through the open doors of the big room where we were gathered. Outside, a broad wooden deck lay bright in the sun, bounded by a dense mass of cypress and by a light iron fence through which was visible the distant meeting of sea and sky.

On this morning, Charlotte had been working on coming to quiet in the eyes and on sensing breathing. For many of us, breathing dominated consciousness. We sat in rapt attention, almost oblivious to sounds from the kitchen and to the passing of occasional curious strollers across the deck.

After perhaps a half hour of such quiet working, Charlotte asked us to lie down. I was reluctant to interrupt. Others also, as I learned later, felt they could have continued such a practice longer. But her good judgment was apparent when I felt myself gratefully accepting the support of the floor along my length.

We lay resting a few minutes and then, at Charlotte's behest, sat up in a circle. In the center of the floor had appeared a small platter of shelled almonds and a bowl of oranges.

Charlotte was all smiles. With the joy of a hostess, she went over to the platter, took it from the floor, and offered an almond to everyone. Some, at the mercy of old reflexes, ate theirs immediately. Others held it in their fingers, or smelled or nibbled. To those whose almond was already gone when she had finished the round, Charlotte offered another, this time with the caution not to eat it yet. An air of expectancy filled the room.

"Can you feel the weight of the almond in your hand?" Charlotte asked, when she had replaced the platter on the floor and sat down herself. After the delicacy of our previous work this morning, it really seemed we could.

"How close must you bring it to your nose to be able to smell it?"

Everywhere among the group were visible expressions of interest.

"What can you feel of the inside of your mouth?" Amused smiles; here and there the half-perceptible movement of a swallow. The saliva was already flowing. Charlotte was like a little girl holding a goodie just out of reach of a dog, teasing it. She was exploiting the magic of contact to the full, and yet, with all her tantalizing, she was working very seriously with consciousness.

"Can you feel your teeth? . . . Your tongue?"

"Try the almond," said Charlotte. "But tastingly! What happens to it after it enters your mouth?"

I could feel the half almond I had bitten off being crushed between my teeth and mingling with my saliva. The faint spice of its initial flavor disappeared, leaving a strange, almost bitter residue. I was not sure I liked it. Indeed, it was usurping consciousness; it was becoming an intrusion.

"How long can you taste it?" Charlotte asked.

Though the taste had changed from its first savor to something quite different, it had not diminished. I wished it would. Furthermore, I was not ready to swallow. Swallowing didn't just happen, as it had always seemed to. It was waiting for an act of will. I took the other half of the almond, and as I began to chew, the thin paste already there, with a curious, half-volitional reflex of the larynx, slipped off into my interior.

"Please raise your hand when you have finished eating," Charlotte said to us. Slowly, after quite a period, hands began to rise. It was several minutes before the last stragglers joined with the rest.

"How would you like to eat like that all the time?"

Expressions of astonishment, even of incredulity, were now voiced among the group. "It would certainly cut down the grocery bills!" someone observed.

No one had suspected that an activity we had repeated so many thousands of times contained such a possibility of new experience. For me, what I had assumed was the taste of an almond had to be discarded as a superficial outer covering, leaving my true sensory connection with it something yet to be explored. If there was a "natural" taste and a "natural" moment in the process of chewing in which the incorporation of this foreign body into me happened by itself, I had never yet felt it out. What might it do for digestion and nourishment if I did?

When the comparisons and discussion had subsided, we slapped ourselves lightly all over. Then Charlotte asked people to take the oranges, start to peel them, and pass them to others who would continue the peeling. As thumbs and finger-nails dug into the thick rinds with varying success, a pungent, bittersweet aroma spread in the air. The oranges passed from hand to hand, each person retaining the fragment of peel he had removed. Then, finally stripped, they were split and resplit until all of the thirty odd people present had at least one seg-ment, as well as one bit of peel. The fragrance of the fruit and sharp bouquet of the rind were perceptible to all.

"Does the odor come to you," Charlotte asked, "when you just allow it to? Or must you sniff it?"

The predatory mien which had been induced in a number of the group by the preparation of the oranges relaxed a little and became more meditative. Eyes softened, expressions quieted.

"What happens when you bring it closer?"

Again I seemed to become all nose and mouth. Contrary to the experience with the almond, the presence of the orange was very strong. Saliva welled around my tongue and through my teeth.

"What happens when you bite into it?"

This bite was more complicated. The skin momentarily resisted my teeth and then broke, the juice spurting in my mouth. In the sweetness was a hint of sourness, and as I now chewed it the delicate flavor faded among the various textures of pulp and skin. Reducing this unequal mixture to a consistency that my gullet would accept, I became suddenly conscious of the equivalence between my own teeth and saliva and the teeth I had seen dripping in dogs and grinding in horses. These teeth were truly made for rending and destroying. But just as truly they were designed to prepare organized tissue for its next stage of life.

It was a joyous and serious occasion. When we had finished, a paper bag was passed around into which each morsel of refuse was dropped in full awareness. Charlotte finally received and set down the bag, ending the class. She bowed slightly with palms together, as is the practice in Zen, and the rest of us bowed almost involuntarily in response. She had found a way of bringing consciousness to what, next to breathing, is the most everyday of all activities, which is at the same time perhaps the central mystery: the passage of life from one form to another.

It was indeed merely another facet of "Meditation in Everyday Living," or giving attention to what we are constantly doing anyhow. But several times, when I have met participants afterward, this has been the experience they remembered most vividly.

■   The scope of sensory awareness can well be illustrated by a contrast between the morning class which I have just described and the class led by me that same afternoon. This class had its beauty and interest too, but in a basic, if perhaps subtle way, it clearly departed from the realm of perception and entered that of symbolism and philosophy. In this crucial respect, the following description differs from all others in this book. I set it down not at all as just another description of the work, but as an example of the kind of deviation from plain sensing which is all too tempting to many others besides myself.

In the afternoon, as I have said, it was my turn to conduct. The slopes at Esalen are covered with aromatic shrubs and trees: sagebrush, pines, cypress, and eucalyptus. I prepared two or three trays, and we offered leaves and twigs to one another to smell. The class flowed very naturally from the morning experiments in tasting, only now everyone also became a host and a guest, a giver and a receiver.

Finally we went out on the deck. Salt air rose gently from sea to mountains. From the slope just above, a host of California poppies glowed down on us. We walked over, and each picked one. Returning to the deck, we stood a moment with eyes closed, feeling the stem of the poppy in our fingers, sensing the faint fragrance borne in on breathing. Quietly, we allowed our eyelids to open. From our own fingers, the golden cup of the flower opened on us like a sunrise.

But it was not only a fine spring day in a lovely setting. It was Good Friday, the last day of our workshop but the first day of the Easter weekend. The urge to preach, even though without words, overcame me. It was to these facts of the calendar, and

Does the odor come to you when you just allow it to?

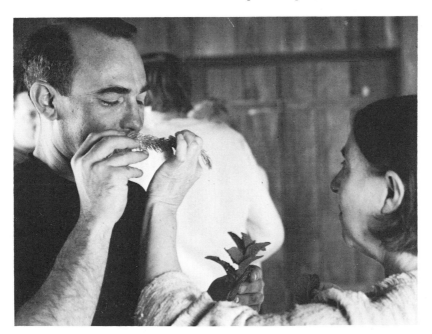

all the emotional values associated with them, that I addressed my next actions. These, as will be readily seen, were not based on experience, either past or present, but on strictly philosophical considerations—a fact which remains unaltered by the additional fact that I managed to embody these considerations in vivid sensory experience.

We stood for some time where we were, gazing into the flowers in our hands, and then I asked each person to crush his flower, seeing and feeling the changes as this form in full bloom was reduced to a speck of almost colorless pulp. We walked slowly to the bank and tossed the remains of our flower into the vegetation. Again we closed our eyes, and after a moment allowed them to reopen. From the bank the multitude of poppies glowed at us.

A child might have asked, why crush a flower for no reason? But I was no child, and neither, I thought, were the participants in the workshop. Yet as we returned, all I could think of was to ask the group if they could *give up thinking* and just give their attention to the changes in the environment. Barefoot, we stepped from the cool earth to the hot, flat boards of the deck and entered the room, whose walls shut out the sea, the flowering slopes, and the breeze, defining the space that was now only there for us. Here too, where smells and sights were so reduced, was still floor to stand on, air to breathe, and the living centers of perception and function which were we.

After what was probably for many people a confusing detour into a private symbolism of the Crucifixion, I began now trying to invite us back to our senses, from which Charlotte never had departed.

26 THE CONNOISSEUR

These experiments with tasting and smelling led me to certain recognitions. After the change in flavor of the almond and the orange, it became obvious, for one thing, how much of what I had considered taste was volatile and actually smell. Of course, I had often heard this said, but now it became experience. I had taken a step, in this modest respect, toward becoming a connoisseur.

I began to experiment more consciously with flavors. With oranges, it became clear that, apart from their fragrance, what was pleasant to me was almost entirely a factor of sweetness—granted that this sweetness was always given character by a certain acidity. With shelled almonds, taste was scarcely a factor at all: I enjoyed the faint aroma as I crushed them, but mainly just the way they crunched between my teeth. Once chewed, they were of no interest.

It became apparent also that taste and smell—which animals, notwithstanding their preferences, seem to use more for identification than for pleasure—have less and less function in a world where more and more foods are processed and labeled. Few people today have occasion to smell whether something is fresh, as was commonly done before the days of refrigerators, quick freezing, and mass processing; and though a great many doubtful smells may have disappeared from the larder, an equal number of delicious smells have disappeared with them. Flavors, which were once a matter of every individual's research, are coming to be adjudicated by computers, which have neither taste buds nor judgment.

But with each child born, a whole new possibility begins.

My own standards of taste go back consciously more than fifty years. I have seldom had peaches or blackberries to match those I picked then. This is not just the enchantment lent by distance, for I remember Spanish oranges in 1934, an Italian persimmon in 1937, apricots from a friend's tree in California in 1947, and even a German pork chop in 1930, just as an old Burgundian may remember wines. These events are memorable for a very real reason: I seldom get fruit that someone has picked because it looked and smelled just right.

In my childhood I heard a good deal about "acquired tastes," meaning adult refinements that the naïve taste buds of a child could not appreciate. But in my travels later among the earthy working people of Latin countries, I seem to remember nothing prized by adults—except, perhaps, alcohols—that was not also prized by children. There, food was food, and good food was good food.

A perfect example of acquired taste is the taste for tobacco, which, of course, is not taste at all, but smell. I gave up smoking many years ago, after a quarter-century of convincing myself that cigarettes tasted as the advertisements said they did; and the one or two I have smoked since then have had the very same nauseating quality they had when I first struggled manfully with them at the age of twelve. I had been told then that cigarettes were bad for me, and was already well aware that much of what was supposed to be bad must really be good, inasmuch as most of the grownups plainly found it so. Conversely, much that was "good for me" was obviously bad. In this, my experience was the same as Tom Sawyer's and I suppose that of many millions of my countrymen. Unfortunately, such a beginning requires a lifetime to correct—a luxury not everyone can afford.

In the world of taste of my childhood there were two universally acknowledged horrors: castor oil and cod-liver oil. Everyone my age had to take them: castor oil as a remedy for stomach-ache, but usually with much emphasis on the folly that had caused the stomach-ache; and cod-liver oil for "good health," but with equal emphasis on the general rule that good was achieved only through suffering. My young friends and I, whatever "good" we came by, were soon resigned to the inevitability of the bad.

A generation later, life brought startling revelations about both my old enemies. The first came when my own child was prescribed percomorph oil. This was administered by the drop instead of by the spoonful, being many times more potent than the oil of my own experience. But it was even more unpleasant, as I found on trying it, and once in one's mouth, the taste hung on and on. Yet when our child was offered it, he took it with delight. In our little progressive nursery school, almost all the children liked percomorph oil, and many would savor it like a *bon vivant* sipping wine. What was the reason? Simply that the oil had been offered them like anything else, and never urged on them.

The other revelation came when I first saw Robert Flaherty's beautiful documentary film, *Nanook of the North*, the pioneer in its field. At the trading post on Hudson Bay, on one of the days when the white man's treasures arrived and were sold, a little Eskimo boy of six had stuffed himself with candies till he felt sick. Fortunately, relief was close at hand. An enormous spoonful of castor oil was poured and brought to his lips. He opened; the spoon was gently advanced; he drew in the thick liquid a little at a time. In my seat, I braced myself against empathy. But even as I could feel the oil spreading over his tongue and filling his nostrils, an expression dawned in his face that unfolded into unforgettable delight. Whatever happened to his sickness, and to the offending candies, at least for the minute that the camera was on him all ill was out of mind and life was good.

English lacks the distinction between the two kinds of *knowing* of Latin languages: between the savant, whose mind is full of information, and the connoisseur, who knows the world as one knows a person. The savant is a man of learning, the connoisseur a man of discrimination. The former has accumulated a world of other people's sometimes doubtful facts, the latter a world of his own sensory experiences.

A former student of Charlotte's had the insight and presence of mind to capture the expressions of the baby shown on these pages. In the glass, in the first group, is the familiar orange juice. The totality of inner preparation for the experience, the total reception, and the full savoring and tasting out show, with that fine clarity of infancy, the process of allowing oneself time and occasion to come to know something, as knowing is implied in the French word *connoisseur*. The photos in the second group tell a different story. At what point in life does "knowledge" begin to separate into these two categories of information and experience? Probably in the midst of one of those many situations for which a million years of evolution have already prepared me, when I am nevertheless told for the first time, "Mother knows best."

One can taste out such photographs just as the baby himself tastes out the juice. One will need much more time than the baby needs, and equal quiet. We have stereotyped reactions that must be put aside, if we are to discover what is there: the presence, the alertness, the sensitivity. There is nothing "cute" about these pictures. For beneath the stereotypes, far beneath, is where we exist ourselves—present, alert, sensitive —when we come deep enough. In the baby, we see ourselves *as we have tasted*—as we may taste again. This is the function of art: to reveal life to us through the sense organs of others, which are no different from our own: the taste buds of the baby, the eye of the photographer. The artist only uses his equipment as we have perhaps not yet learned to use ours.

The magic of *taste*, which everyone who knows the word respects, either by compulsion or genuinely, and which commands so high a price on the market of art, design, decoration, and fashion in the United States, is no secret painfully acquired from others. It is the universal and perfectly commonplace magic of our sensory nervous system, at the center of which are the taste buds, constantly discriminating— relishing or rejecting—when they are permitted to, endlessly making fine observations and judgments which are only too often overruled by parents and teachers whose own taste buds have been dulled and whose native discrimination has been superseded by the standards of others. From this simple animal function, which civilization has merely refined and com-

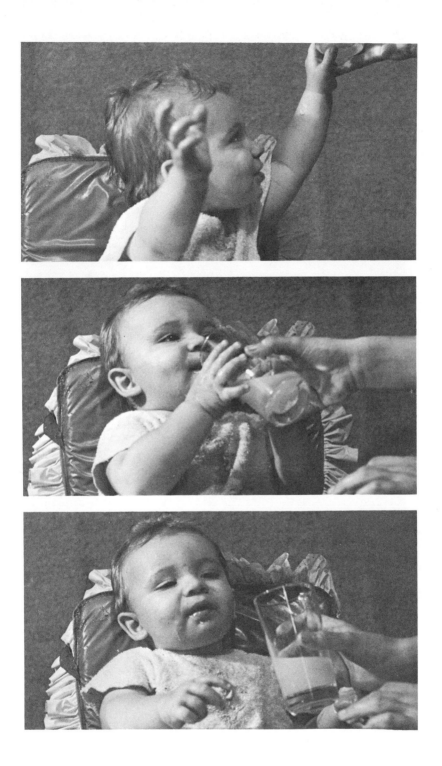

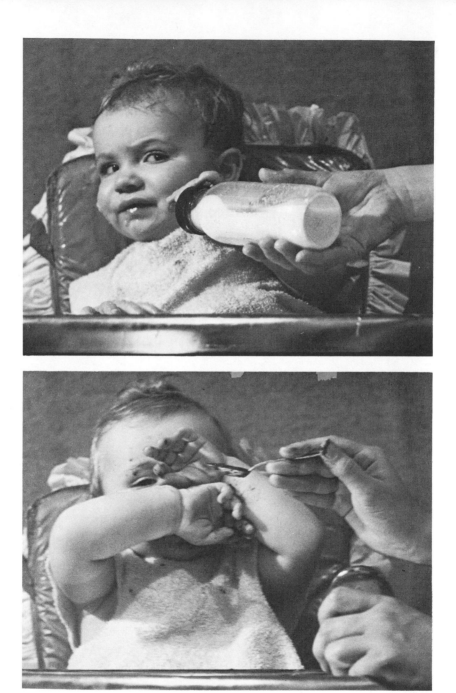

plicated, comes the one word used to denote that judgment of human achievements from which there is no appeal.

It is thus an error to think of connoisseurs as a rare and privileged group of adults who have had the leisure and interest (or do we think of it as time and money?) to spend their lives in fine comparisons of food and drink, and of the arts. No household would be without its connoisseur, if we parents had the good sense to respect him. We would all be connoisseurs ourselves if we only respected our natural gifts. No art-lover sensing out a painting, no lover of music savoring a fine quartet, indeed, no ordinary sensitive person pausing at the song of a bird or relishing a sunset, is differently engaged from a baby tasting his juice when he is just allowed to do so. One cannot be taught to taste, for it comes naturally; one can only be distracted from it.

Would this not explain why every primitive culture produces artifacts of such exquisite form and color? No experts are needed here to point out values which everyone can see for himself.

Our sensory awareness classes exist to cultivate the connoisseur in each of us. But far better, if one had to choose, would be to study and let oneself be influenced by one's own child. Such a study would mean giving up one's preconceptions and taking whatever time might be needed to come to know the child's way of being. One who could do this would, I think, truly become a connoisseur of living.

27 YAWNING AND STRETCHING

A nother thing babies can teach us is how to yawn. Whoever has not really seen a baby yawn—or, indeed, still better, a cat or dog—has missed a full organismic experience. When I first attended Charlotte's classes in New York, and for the first time was encouraged not to hide a yawn but to permit and enjoy it, I became painfully conscious of the very limited degree to which yawning was still possible to me. The impulse came often enough, but each time it seemed like a bud starting to open in all promise and then mysteriously blighted. There was the opening of jaws and throat, the intake of breath, and then, as neck and shoulder girdle began to become involved, came an abrupt ending, as with a boat starting to drift in the breeze and stopped short by its anchor. It began so sweetly and was so rudely halted. Struggle was futile. I seemed to stand impotent on the edge of opening. (The sexual connotations of these statements, especially for women, seem to me so obvious that I shall proceed without further mention of them.)

Once I asked Charlotte if she thought we New Yorkers could ever learn to yawn like dogs and cats. Her reply was immediate and Delphic: "Dogs and cats are also New Yorkers." This was a hard message to take, but I have pondered it and pass it on.

The firm hand on my shoulder which arrested the budding yawn within was the hand of a form of law and order which, though absent from many cultures, is highly developed in ours. We conceal our yawns not only because they sometimes express boredom, or because we are ashamed of admitting sleepiness, but also because not to conceal them would reveal a yielding to the involuntary which our social rules can hardly sanction. In fact, we commonly speak of "suppressing" and even "stifling" yawns—as one does with an insurrection.

But if we would accept and take heed of our need to yawn, it could become a very reliable safety valve and guide, giving us the clue when it is time to start afresh and come to a better balanced activity, or a more genuine communication, as the case might be. When everyone in a situation recognized the authenticity of a yawn, we could have a good yawn, or a good laugh, all around.

Laughing is in a sense the other side of the coin. It is a celebration of survival and well-being, whether alone or with others, in a world of perils and absurdities. Yawning and laughter, as everybody knows, are equally contagious, and are two of the best lifeboats we can share on our long voyage.

We shall no more attempt to work directly with yawning than we should with laughing or weeping or making love. These basic reflexes, like "the truth," can be approached only indirectly. We shall work on our house to have it ready for them, in case they should visit us, but they belong to a deeper order of things than our ideas and intentions, and they will not stand urging or improving.

There is, however, an activity very closely related to yawning, and even to a certain extent including it, which represents a kind of general and universal aspiration toward freedom, and which almost everybody already works with who concerns himself with "movement." This is *stretching*, in which lions, wolves, and babies are as eloquent as in their yawns. Who has not noticed the relish and power with which a cat stretches and bares its claws, or the gusto of a dog stretching limbs and back before arising? We, too, on waking in the morning, while our minds are still half in that world we cannot aspire to control, and we still smell of sleep, often spontaneously stretch out of the position we have lain in, savoring our flexibility and extension to the full and involuntarily readying ourselves for a new day.

As with lying, however, we shall probably have to work on stretching before it can become restful to us again when we are wide awake. Very many of us have been taught how to stretch—

as though there could be a correct *method* for this simplest and most spontaneous of all expressive movements. We must start in an entirely different way. We must first come to enough inner quiet so that we can feel what may really be needed at this moment. Then stretching will become discovery and not performance, a meditation instead of an exercise. When we have come closer to real stillness, in which we can feel the very beginning of a movement, we will let it begin at its own time and then follow it as it evolves and gains power, leading us on its own path into virgin territory, where no experts have been.

To stretch with subtlety and sensitivity.

This highly intuitive stretching, which would only be a conscious equivalent of a process which simply happens in babies
and animals (but which we could never find by a mechanical
imitation of babies or animals), can be practiced by anyone at
any time, even when among other people. Much of what one
can feel of oneself is so hidden from sight that it can move and
stretch itself unnoticed. In fact, it is well worth trying when
among others. One is then obliged to stretch with subtlety and
sensitivity—a practice which will also prove its worth when one
is alone, or working on stretching with a group, when one
might be tempted to go into all sorts of exaggerations. Such,
exaggerations blur the distinction between what is actually
sensed as needed (and can be allowed), and what one imagines
is needed, and brings about by force. A stretch that extends
itself only as the tissues invite it, and does not force its way
through, becomes an awakening for proper functioning and
brings genuine well-being.

I believe the reader can obtain much relief and pleasure if
he will take ten or fifteen minutes once in a while just to
explore stretching. I would suggest standing as a point of departure, though any other will do. It can and should be practiced
as a real meditation: that is, as something to which one gives
full and unreserved attention. To fling oneself here and there
in an image of "abandon," as many people do, or to relax everything possible in an image of "letting go," is as much a form of
self-control as following any other pattern of behavior. It may
be satisfying, just as it is satisfying to feel that one has done the
correct steps of a tango, or has jumped loosely to rock and roll;
but just as merely doing the steps is not dancing, this "abandon"
should by no means be confused with the sensitive feeling out of
oneself which is spontaneous movement.

Each moment the reader will really give himself to his discoveries will be a memorable one. As in all meditations,
strength and patience are required, for the voices of the past
will be clamoring to have their way: the advice, the techniques,
the examples of people one has seen and admired. It is hard to
shut these voices out and wait in the unfamiliar emptiness
until the organism speaks its needs. But one must hold firm to

the emptiness and wait for this voice, which can always be recognized because it never commands or urges, but says merely, "I am here." One can recognize it by the pleasure one has in hearing it—and in allowing the hand to open and extend, if it is the hand, or the sacrum if it is the sacrum, or the jaw and windpipe if it is a yawn, or little by little the whole organized skeleton and musculature, if it should lead so far.

28 REACHING AND SERVING

Another closely related practice in our classes is reaching. However much or little we yawn and stretch, reaching is something we are constantly obliged to do in daily living. What we are not obliged to do is to reach wholeheartedly—like the people in these pictures—and we seldom do.

Now if we sit cross-legged on the floor with a stone lying a little away from us, we cannot reach for it without the movement's bringing our trunk and hip joints into play. Even the muscles of our legs will be asked to give. It may be necessary to make a conscious choice: either to remain as inert as the situation permits—perhaps even straining ourselves to avoid unnecessary motion—or to accept the invitation to a more total response. This is clearly not a mechanical problem, but a psychosomatic one. It is a question of attitude.

Perhaps we are just asked to pick up the stone. One single task, as spoken or written, and a single task if given to a machine. But proposed to twenty people, it elicits twenty different responses. One person is eager to obey, another is reluctant, one aggressive, another diffident, one light, another heavy. To at least some degree, the individual mood and character of each is apparent in the movement.

All, however, share the relative mechanical difficulty of reaching out while sitting cross-legged on the floor. Our basic choice, regardless of our individual differences, is whether to perform the minimum which is literally required of us or whether, in addition, to feel out what we are doing. Nothing is gained by just picking up the stone, but to sense how we go about it may bring valuable discoveries. This may bring into

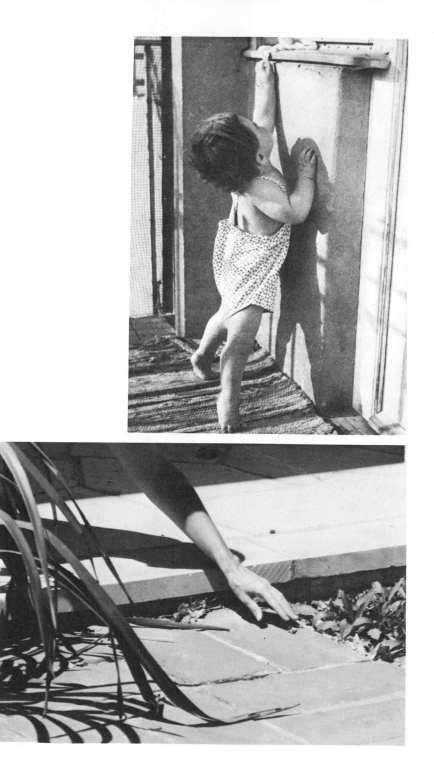

relief how little accustomed we are to yield where we would have to in order to reach freely, without constriction all through our interior. It may dawn on us that for years we have performed such tasks in spite of ourselves, so to speak—forcing ourselves, even if only briefly, and straining back and belly against increasing resistance in pelvis and legs.

Faced with such a choice, some of us will begin to reach for our stone with a deliberate stretching and exercising of the pelvis, such as is often done in dance exercises and in yoga. Now comes the question already discussed,[1] to what extent we will allow ourselves to be led away from the task of *reaching freely for the stone* into a mechanical forcing of sluggish muscles so as to become more limber. This is a very delicate and subtle question. At its simplest, I would say the alternative is between following the *idea* of a correct reaching, in which one simply trains oneself as one might a dog, and taking time to explore where one could yield more fully, as a living, breathing organism, to a given task.

This alternative may not really exist as we begin. We may have to start with what I am again calling "exercise." But as soon as we have started, the alternative does appear, and the two possibilities presently become clearer and more separate. As in all our practice, the way of exploration becomes constantly more distinct from the way of authority.

But the reader need not sit cross-legged on the floor to experiment with reaching. Before he sets down the book or reaches for the lamp, let him give attention to his own breathing until he feels where it goes in him and perhaps where it would still like to go more freely. Then as he reaches out for whatever purpose, he may go slowly enough to sense how the movement affects him, and how possibly a more generous and open movement might influence breathing. This, in turn, will affect the way he picks up or sets down whatever is involved, regardless of its weight.

We are constantly reaching during the day while standing or walking: opening and closing doors, selecting and replacing

1. See page 69.

articles, pressing elevator buttons, shaking hands. Above all, the housewife is involved in reaching when she cooks and serves—or the househusband, as is often the case with Charlotte and me. He may be setting a full pan on the stove or reaching out to get plates from a shelf. Or he may be placing a dish on the dining table, where the important thing is its relationship to all the other plates and to the people. It was in the instantaneous, unthinking, and perfect resolution of all these matters by our Los Angeles cook, in which he allowed himself to be equally and totally involved throughout his person, that his great beauty lay.

I would advise anyone who is interested in either movement or social relations to get a job as a waiter. Half the fine dancers I have known have earned a living as waiters or waitresses. Kinesthetically, it is the perfect occupation. But he should go either to a lunch counter in midtown Manhattan, where at noon every second is weighed in gold, or, conversely, to some remote Savoyard village, where the food comes from the garden and from the stream outside the back door of the restaurant, and is precious to him who prepares it and to him who eats it. For no waiter can be entirely free of the brutish and alienated attitude to the ritual of eating that prevails in so many American restaurants. Unless he is reminded by circumstances of the intrinsic value of his work, he can hardly give himself to it with all his heart.

But for the sensitive waiter, in a milieu where there is respect for this most basic of all organic processes, in which one form of life is prepared for and consumed by another, his work becomes full sensory awareness. Its intrinsic social and individual significance is probably why, in good restaurants all over the world, the waiter wears the simplest possible costume of white and black, representing cleanliness and unobtrusiveness and allowing psychological freedom. What shall we say of what America does to her own waitresses, dressing them in miniskirts and even baring their breasts to distract us and them from their real function?

We cannot all become professional waiters and waitresses. But I wonder if the reader has not himself felt now and then a certain exhilaration in serving his friends, his children, or his mate. If so, was it just the joyful sense of offering a gift— perhaps the work of his own hands—and of setting the gift down before the recipient? Or was there still another element, the joy of movement, which was equally present when he removed the dishes and carried them to the sink—with care, in respect for the others' presence, but perhaps swiftly and efficiently nonetheless. Here there was a choice of dumping them at random—of giving up and letting go, one might say —or of addressing oneself intuitively and unhesitatingly to the situation, sorting and scraping here, perhaps rinsing there, without ever neglecting the company at the table. If one has had this experience, was there not a very satisfying sense of functioning in it?

Perhaps when he next sets the table or carries dishes to the sink, the reader will make a deliberate experiment for himself. He may take time to sense his own breathing as he moves, or to feel the weight and shape of the objects he handles. What if he merely gives attention to his own relation to the floor in moving, or to his passage through the spaces of the room? These avenues of sensing can be interchangeable. All such activities, involving the placing and removing of objects in accordance with a sense of the entire situation, requiring mindfulness but seldom requiring thought, can be studied just as one studies reaching for a stone.

Would this not lead to an unbearable narcissism in serving others, when hungry people might wait while we perfect our movements? By no means. Does gravity wait while a skier perfects his style? All our actions, if functional, are directed to the central aim of the moment—in this case, serving nourishment to others. In such a light, studying will not diminish one's connection with other people present, but can only enhance it.

29   GIVING AND RECEIVING

Having practiced with inanimate objects, we may begin again working with other people, more mindful now of what is really involved. There is so much to learn about another through conscious contact, and especially through what is called "physical" contact—through the open, sensitive coming into connection, even through clothes, with the flesh and blood of another person. I say "even through clothes," but I have felt it through the twenty-foot length of a floor beam, when one end of the beam was on my shoulder and the other on my partner's, as we walked out on twelve-inch walls, high above the ground, to set the beam in place. Unless each feels the other through the length of such a beam, neither survives. A contact of skin with skin may be delightful, but the deep inner nature of a person must come *through* the skin, and it will come through the clothes too.

One year, I spent half an hour or so every afternoon wrestling with my five-year-old son when I came home from heavy work in the shipyards. It was a delight for him and a great restorative for me. His friends began to join in, until on occasion there might be quite a group of us. It was an extraordinary discovery for me how clearly each child's character became apparent through the veils of behavior with which I was already familiar, already so strongly formed at that early age: one joyous and generous in his use of force, one sly and relentless, one anxious, one fearful and mean—each test of strength more revealing than months of everyday encounter. The opinions I had formed of them could be discarded, for in wrestling I felt that I came to know each little boy as he really was—behind the social façade he had learned at home—and as he might never know himself.

In our experiments, which so far have only skirted wrestling, something of this may still appear with adults. The forces beneath the surface make themselves felt. A shy person may have a warm and positive approach, while a big talker may be timid and awkward. One who acts self-confident and omniscient may be helpless in real action. Experts on sensitivity may be cold, experts in expressive dance exaggerated. Someone who feels and appears incompetent in the stresses of social

Our experiments, which so far have only skirted wrestling.

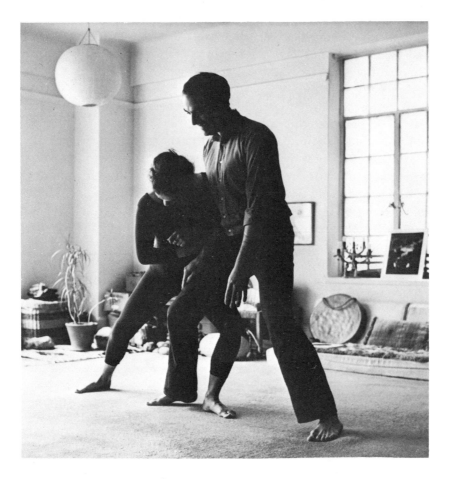

living may, on the other hand, really come into his own when he works quietly with another person. Careful perception of what actually happens may teach us much about the discrepancy between surface appearance and inner reality.

Real human relationships consist of constant exchange. Consciously or unconsciously, one is always giving and receiving. Sometimes it seems more one or more the other, and sometimes both simultaneously. Actually, in a sense it is always both at once. A warm hand and a cold hand come together: the one gives of its warmth, and the other receives. But the cold hand gives an invitation to the warmth, and the warm hand receives the invitation. Either may be reluctant and hold back, or be accepting and give freely. One gives the other a glass of wine, but the recipient gives the giver the occasion. The guest gives the host a better or poorer reception for the meal he is given. One cannot separate these functions; one can only be more or less present in them.

Ways of working together are innumerable. When it fully dawns on one that this work is indeed not a body of techniques but the exploration of a new approach to living, new ways appear like the new leaves in spring, spontaneously, from the situation itself. But some activities are so well suited to a studio, and so general and dramatic in their usual effects, that I should like to describe them here.

One interesting study, which could easily be tried by the reader and his friends as a sort of parlor game, is to explore what happens when one person stands and others offer to support his arms. Three people work together, one standing alone with arms extended to the sides, while the other two stand behind him ready to offer their support. When all feel ready, the two bring their hands under the elbows and wrists of the other, who is invited to give them the weight of his arms. He is not to lean on the helpers. He is to let his arms be carried, but in all other respects to stand normally.

The helpers, meanwhile, stand patiently offering a support which of course they cannot give until the other first gives his weight. When, in their judgment, they are receiving all or most of the weight of the other's arms, they may move them gently here and there, feeling whether the other lets them do the moving, or resists, or perhaps tries to do it himself. Finally the helpers carry the arms down until they come to hanging and, when they feel they are no longer needed, come quietly away.

Very often, at one point or another, a helper may feel his offer of support is not accepted. He may want to say so, or he may wait quietly, just staying there. After a while, if still no weight is given, he may deftly withdraw, leaving the arm, which presumably was resting in his hands, to remain magically outstretched, unfelt by the person himself until his attention is brought to it. This is most apt to happen when the arm is being lowered, but often no weight is ever given at all.

People are almost always impressed with their discoveries in this experiment. But what is significant is the changes that may take place, from not giving to giving, or vice versa, whether noticed by one, two, or all three parties concerned. One very cultivated and intelligent woman who has worked with us for a number of years without losing much of her obviously rigorous self-control exclaimed recently in delight, "This is the first time I could really give myself." When her partners were asked how

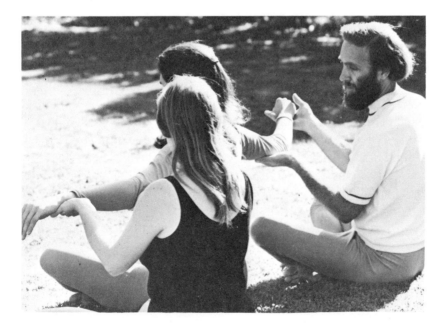

it felt to them, both agreed that she had not given any weight at all. She was quite taken aback, but then conceded that she had not given herself *at first*. "But when I felt I could trust them," she said, smiling warmly with moist eyes, "then I gave." The partners, asked to reconsider carefully, did remember that each, at a certain point, seemed to feel more contact. How much weight was involved they could not tell: certainly not much. But it was true there had been a change.

It would be hard to find a clearer example of the relativity of experience. The few ounces which seemed nothing to the helpers were, to the person who granted them, the first stone loosening in the wall, which seemed to her like a landslide. As the greatest sinners were the most welcomed in heaven, the person with the greatest stone wall between himself and the world may find the most delight as one after another, in their own time, the stones begin to slip away.

No matter how fully or how little one is able to give of oneself, the least yielding of one's arms to another in rest, and even more when they are being moved, is perceived as freedom —often as weightlessness and even flight. People come back to standing as from a magic carpet, exhilarated and softened. They are grateful to the ones who gave the help, and in the contagion of exchange the helpers are grateful too.

When a group can be divided into units of four, six, or eight, another vivid experiment can be made in giving and receiving. Half—let us say four of eight—will stand holding hands in a circle. The other four will sit or kneel behind them, one behind each. The four who stand take time to come to a good distribution of their weight and an easy connection with each other. Then, using each other's hands for balance, they raise their heels from the floor, coming to standing on the balls of their feet. The helpers at this point quietly slip their hands under the raised heels, which are now offered a very different support to return to. Those who stand are asked to come gradually back to easy standing, with the balls of the feet on the floor and heels and insteps on their helpers' hands. The helpers, who, if prudent, have removed their rings, are to speak up if it hurts; otherwise, those standing are to give their full weight. When they feel they have indeed come to standing on what is under them, they are to rise again, allowing the helpers to withdraw, and find how the floor feels now when they come back to it.

While they are feeling out what is usually a fresher and livelier connection with the floor, the helpers move a quarter of the way around the circle to the next person, who presently rises again with his comrades to allow the new helper's hands to slip under him. With four standing and four helping, each has three new opportunities for readjustment and fresh approach, in which he can explore the best way to offer his hands or to give his weight to another without crushing him.

Afterward, when all compare their findings, it is sometimes the heaviest who are felt as lightest, and the lightest as heaviest. Only part of this discrepancy is due to fear of crushing the other; much is in the way the weight is given. A rigid person either does not give his weight at all or gives it rigidly in the form of pressure, which will probably also be true of a less sensitive person. But helpers who wring crushed fingers after their first offering may find their way to a quite different and perhaps much fuller approach as they continue, and one much less painful.

Far oftener, however, helpers find that they can take much more of the other's weight than they imagined, and that they experience it not as an imposition on the part of the other, but as a giving which they find pleasure in accepting. The givers also, who can choose how much weight to give to the floor and how much to their partners' hands, gradually come to more and more standing on the offered hands and are amazed both at the capacity of the hands to receive them and at the sensitivity in their own feet which can tell them whether they are giving or imposing.

In the chapter on lying, I described the experiment of raising one's legs to standing and then slightly raising the pelvis from the floor in order to explore what may be a long way back to rest.[1] This same experiment, when undertaken with a partner, gains an added liveliness. When the pelvis is raised, the partner

1. See pages 72-73.

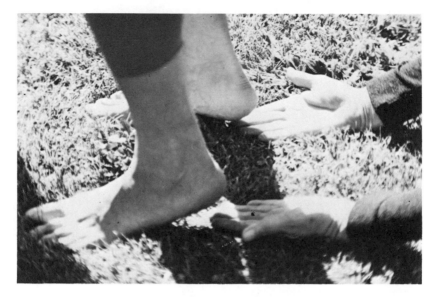

Helpers who wring crushed fingers after their first offering
may find their way to a much fuller approach
as they continue.

slips his hand underneath to receive it when it is allowed down
to rest.

So much that is movable, and so much often unrealized
sensitivity, reside in the lowest part of the back, matching the
flexibility and sensitiveness of the hand, that the coming into
union may be very fully felt and savored, and the very considerable weight given and received, without injury or even stress.
And when the pelvis is again raised to free the helper's hand
and again finds its way, perhaps now with every nerve awake,
to the flat and solid floor, the yielding that is asked of it and
the support that is offered may have gained very much in
reality and value.

30 GIVING AND RECEIVING, CONTINUED

One of the best ways of getting a group into a sense of interconnection is simply to let them exchange objects with each other. As Charlotte and I are seldom without stones, which we even take on planes and through customs, these are what we often use for this purpose. The exchanges in our classes have this great advantage over the exchange of Christmas presents that our gifts are temporary, cost nothing, and are unfailingly beautiful.

We have only to ask participants to stay in touch with the stone in their hand as they give it over to another person for the exchange to become significant. Something real is passing from one person to the other, and the manner of its passing is entirely dependent on the two people concerned. When aware of the stone, one also feels the other receiving it. The receiver, for his part, may be conscious of how the stone is given— whether with care and feeling, or otherwise. When I say "care and feeling," I do not mean concern and affection, though it is quite possible these emotions may be generated as a consequence. I mean the maintaining of interest in the transaction until it is completed: feeling when it *is* completed—when form and weight have been fully transferred to the receiving hand— and withdrawing at the appropriate moment without hurry or reluctance. All this can be felt by the receiver. He, too, feels the weight of the stone as it is given to him, and he feels whether it is simply the weight and nothing else, or perhaps includes some additional little push—as if the giver wanted to get rid of his stone, or impress him with it—or some unwillingness to leave, as if the giver clung to it.

One or two questions to the class may be helpful. For

instance, do people really just stay with the transfer of the stones, or do they little by little become carried away in self-image and fantasy? Are their movements, however sensitive, also simple and practical, or do they become gestures?

In order to facilitate exchange, we usually ask everybody to walk at random through the room until he feels an impulse to give away his stone and receive another. The use of the eyes immediately comes into question. Do I look for a suitable person for my exchange? Perhaps there is some other way of sensing him. How can I tell whether he also is ready to exchange? Instead of the usual questioning and answering with glances, is there a way of revealing my desire and sensing his simply through kinesthetic awareness? As these possibilities begin to arise for people in the group, the whole activity becomes quiet and charged with alertness. When the encounter occurs, growing into the exchange and consummated by it, care and feeling blossom into a greater sense of presence. Again we are expanded to our potential: able to *be*, without reflection—able simply and fully to exchange.

In our New York studio we have many beautiful stones for such uses, just the size for our hands. But we have large ones too—ten or twenty-pounders from Wyoming, California, Canada, Mexico. One stone, like the egg of a roc out of the *Arabian Nights*, brought to us from Nova Scotia, weighs sixty pounds. With this stone, marvelously rounded by North Atlantic storms, it is a joy to work on lifting. This is my hobby. I ask someone just to bend over and clasp this stone—to let its smooth ends fill his hands as he stoops to where he can feel it most comfortably—and then gradually to take a little of its weight. As the person works, he is to be sure to accommodate his breathing, to let his back and belly have freedom, and not to strain. In fact, the task is to explore the difference between working and straining. If he wants to take more weight he is free to do so, but under no circumstances is he to lift this really heavy stone from the floor. And yet, even with little old ladies in these New York classes, the stone *does* leave the floor—no one knows how!

The heavier stones, like the smaller ones, were chosen for

their beauty, and they stand in a good light on our window sills as objects of art. Over the years, they have accumulated till there is hardly room for them.

One morning I had the class form a circle and then asked one person to go to the window, take one of these heavy stones from among its surroundings, carry it back to the circle, and give it to the person nearest him. This exchange had to be careful, for if the stone had inadvertently dropped on someone's foot, it might have meant real injury. The recipient, with some concern and doubtfulness, accepted the weight, turned and passed it on cautiously to his neighbor, and finally went himself to the window to get another stone. Soon a number of heavy stones, interspersed with flower pots and other objects, were traveling around the circle—each very different in shape, weight, and character from the others, and each given and received with as much concern for its weight as interest in its individuality. Little by little, doubtfulness disappeared. Standing eased, breathing became freer. When the first stone reached the last person in the circle, that person returned it to its place.

The hour and a half which a New York class takes was soon over. Except for a preparation in sensing with our usual stones, it had been entirely consumed in taking these heavy stones from their places, carrying them over and giving them to the waiting hands and energies of another human being, and, finally, receiving a stone in turn and replacing it where it had come from. At the end of the class, one woman came to me in tears. Through an oversight, she had not been asked either to take a stone from its place or to return it.

■ One night found us working at the other end of the continent, with Charlotte conducting the final session of a San Francisco Zen Center benefit attended by two hundred people. She had been working at sensing breathing while sitting, standing, and coming into movement—an activity especially appropriate to these circumstances in which she could relate the central concern of Zen practice to everyday living. At a certain point she paused, and, in accordance with

careful prearrangement, fifty candles in saucers were brought
into the room. These were then distributed among the people
present and lighted by whoever had matches, until points of
light could be seen flickering on all sides.

The hall was now darkened and each bearer of a candle
asked to walk at random through the crowd until he came to
someone to whom he felt impelled to give it. In the semidark-
ness of the great room, a sea of hushed forms began to move,
opening a little and closing around the wandering lights, while
here and there someone would give his candle to some momentarily illuminated stranger, or receive one from him. Everywhere eyes were on the moving flames, which, flickering,
irregularly as they were carried, yet warmly lighted each
transient encounter that formed and dissolved. Each person
present alternated between the anonymity of the slowly moving, darkened multitude and the moment when the candle was
in his own hands to carry. Accepting so clear a role when it
came to him, and relinquishing it when he felt it was the
moment—feeling out the rightness and inevitability of each
—invited a profound sense of rhythm and seemed to confer on
the faces of the participants a glow beyond that radiating from
the light. Among the two hundred persons milling in the room,
some with lights, some without, spread a gradual exhilaration
that did not seem to diminish as the time passed.

After half an hour, Charlotte asked all those who had candles to set them down in the center of the floor. Even with
these students and others interested in Zen, for whom simplicity is paramount, this process occupied a considerable time.
When it was finished, those nearest the center sat or knelt on
the floor, so that the others, massed behind them, could see over
their heads. Finally, Charlotte asked someone to come forward
and blow out a candle. The room filled with expectancy. In the
corners of their eyes, people could see the ring of figures surrounding the fifty candles, whose flames lighted the banked
faces on every side. A young man arose, his eyes fixed on the
glittering pool of light, and stood an instant, as though taking
heart. Then he walked forward, knelt, blew out the nearest
candle in one breath, and returned to where he had been.

Before everyone's eyes, one of the white candles stood still, tipped only by a small black wick. Finally another figure arose, and from the opposite side still another. The task had begun; hesitation was evaporating. Without haste or confusion, three or four now approached at once, blew out a candle each, and returned to their places. Each moved with the assurance and grace of a deep inner motivation.

Presently only some dozen candles were left. Charlotte struck a small bell she had brought with her. The movements of the figures that were just arising halted as the tone of the bell shivered through the room in gradual diminuendo. At the center of everything, the remaining candles burned steadily. Charlotte stepped forward, brought her palms together in the Zen greeting, and bowed, ending the session.

31 GIVING AND RECEIVING THE HEAD

Of all the more usual ways in which we work together, probably the most dramatic is when we lift one another's heads. In this experiment, one person lies on his back on the floor, while the other sits or kneels behind his head where he can easily reach it. If we have already worked with someone's leg, as described earlier, or supported his arms, we will be prepared for some of the possibilities.

Will our partner entrust his head to us? Will we, for our part, be able to see or feel any of the changes which his reaction to our offer of support may induce in him? Will we be able to feel if we entrust our head to him?

Firstly, we are more concerned now with how we approach the task. We take time to get settled where we shall not be working at a disadvantage. We also wait until our partner signals that he is quiet and ready for us. Then we gently slip our hands under his neck, exploring through the hair to find where neck enters skull: the region where we shall be able to lift the weight of the head securely without a tendency to push it into the trunk.

We allow time to get the feel of the other and to let him get the feel of us. Then we begin to lift. Our eyes are on our partner's whole person. Every change in breathing is visible, every fluctuation in the musculature of throat and chest, every flutter in the eyelids. According to these clear messages we proceed, raising the head a little distance from the floor, supporting it as our partner may or may not become more confident in us, perhaps very gently moving or turning it if he permits. Finally we lower the head until we feel the floor has fully received it and we are no more needed. We leave quietly, as a mother might leave a sleeping baby, with no disturbing farewell.

But this is not the end. For some time, the one lying may continue to feel changes taking place in himself, and some of these may be visible to the helper. Or the thoughts may be so clustering in him that there is no room for sensation; and this too will be visible in his expression.

This experiment is, in fact, apt to stir up so many energies and so much interest that often one has to interrupt animated conversations between partners and ask them to share their discoveries with the group. Most frequently, the question will be, did the lying one yield his head or did he move it himself? With a little reflection, however, much else may come up. Someone may recollect that at the first full contact, before the head was even raised, he felt powerful changes in his connection with the floor. He could accept the invitation to rest in another's hands, and as he did so, he felt his groins open up and his legs come to fuller lying. This openness may still be felt afterward, even after coming up to standing. Another may have felt mainly the fearfulness of being dropped: his partner's hands never seemed secure to him, even when they gripped him. All the possibilities in working with a leg are present here too, with a drama added by the special value we attach to our heads.

One of my most striking recollections of early days in Charlotte's classes was during a weekend seminar when this experiment was tried. On this occasion, it was my own head that was raised; and the hands that raised it seemed so timid, and the whole person behind them so insecure and frail, that it required all my resolution to give my weight. I felt that at any moment I might be dropped, and it was necessary to remind myself that it was only an inch or so down to the floor. As these quavering hands held me, my mind's eye, quite unable to rest, reviewed the thirty figures I had seen in the room, and I decided that my helper must be one of two elderly and seemingly infirm ladies whom I had already noticed. I could not wait, after the attempt was over, to see who it was. My eyes strained backward to the figure kneeling behind me. To my amazement, I saw the outline, and then beyond any doubt the face, of the most jovial and self-confident member of my regular evening class, a one-time college athlete who could still lift a weight equal to his own two hundred pounds, and a leader in his business community.

As I write this, some fifteen years later, it is only two weeks since my head was raised again, on a similar weekend, by hands so gentle and secure, bespeaking a person so confident and strong, that, had there been a Japanese wrestler in the class, I should have been sure it was he. I have learned, in these fifteen years, to stay with sensing and not to wonder or imagine who may be working with me. But after all was over I had an opportunity to see, and so unusual was the impression made on me that I availed myself of it. It was a slim, fragile-looking young girl.

Working with hundreds of such experiments, I have learned that one of the questions that most often occupies participants is whether women and men come through differently as helpers. To me this question has always seemed irrelevant.

We allow time to get the feel of the other.

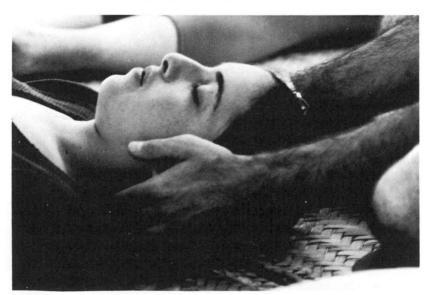

But for those interested, these experiences would be worth considering.

The one who has helped may also report experiences. Quite possibly he noticed changes, shallow or deep, in his partner's breathing. Often it turns out that the partner was unaware of them and, in the latter case at least, when breathing had deepened, remembers only a sensation of security and trust that was very satisfying. Or the helper may have noticed strong pulsations and struggling in his partner's throat, indicating a desire to yield and the anxiety preventing it. In such a case, if he was able more and more quietly, gently, and surely to continue offering support, letting his own pores be open for these signals of response and distress, so that he could feel more sensitively how his help was needed, he may have made possible at last a moment of giving for which the other was filled with a mysterious relief and gratitude. Often, when all went well, the one helped remained lying in a delicious well-being, which he remembers as a new openness for existence inward and outward.

Because of the questions raised by this experiment—the

Then we begin to lift.

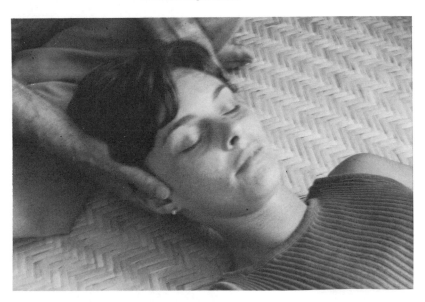

yielding of one's most complex and valued extremity, for most people the very seat of their identity, to the hands of another— this is exciting to everyone. It has become one of the most popular "sensory techniques," and is often used merely for its value as sensationalism. But when worked with sensitively, it is a study demanding much time and care and offering significant rewards.

A useful variation is to require two signals from the person lying: the first when he has come to enough quiet to be ready to begin, and the second when his partner's hands have come into a connection where he feels secure with them, at which point the partner can begin to lift. If, now, the helper is sufficiently aroused and present for the task, the other's head may leave and return to the floor as inevitably and imperceptibly as

---

Lying in a delicious well-being.

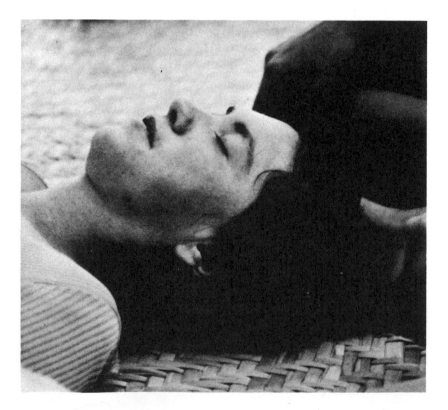

driftwood on a sheltered beach is raised by the incoming tide, buoyed, perhaps moved, for whatever time it is, and then silently given back to the firm sand.

As in raising the legs, a steady, gentle pull on the head—an invitation to give up its clinging to the neck and shoulders—follows naturally when the head is raised from the base of the skull. If this invitation is of such a quality that he can avail himself of it, it will offer an entirely new freedom to the person lying. I believe it takes us back to the time we lay, or at least needed to lie, in our mother's arms. That time may have meant for us feelings ranging anywhere from anxiety to bliss. As with those haunting smells which once in a while speak to us of a time almost before memory, such an occasion as the present one may offer us a taste of the half-forgotten bliss, or a possibility for disinterring and compensating the old anxiety.

To me, in these connections, images of natural forces come readily. I see the tide rise, and I feel some equivalent in myself. Two other such forces speak in that fine fable of Aesop's, which I think could well stand as a maxim for all our work with one another.

The Sun and the North Wind met over some ancient Athenian slope and made a wager as to which of them could soonest get the coat off a traveler walking on the earth below. The North Wind, full of action and purpose, tried first, but the harder he blew the tighter the traveler pulled his coat around him. Finally exhausted, he stopped and allowed the Sun his turn. But the Sun did nothing special; as always, after a storm, in those clear Greek skies, he merely smiled down on the traveler in his full presence. He was still smiling as the traveler walked on coatless down the road and the North Wind blustered off back home.

This kind of presence we can work to cultivate.

32 PLAYING WITH BALLS

I remember that when I first worked with stones in Charlotte's studio I was so enchanted that afterward I could not wait until I had a stone of my own. On each trip to the country I searched until I finally came on one, well rounded and just the right size, that I took home, where it became my companion in action, my pillow, or my burden, as the fancy led me. But if Charlotte has favorite objects, they seem to be balls.

The first problem in working with balls is to survive the explosion of reflexes that tends to follow immediately upon their distribution to a group. For many people, difficult as it is to be quiet and attentive under any circumstances, with a ball in the hand it is impossible. As well ask a dog to be quiet with a bone.

Whereas a stone has a certain silent presence that invites contemplation, a ball asks to be played with. Its shape is geometrical, ideal, and without individuality. Its entire reason for being is action, and this action may be the very giving and receiving which we are studying. So when Charlotte has rolled out a basketful of balls among a group, and each person, having taken one in his characteristic way of taking, now stands there, seeing it and feeling it in his hands—or more likely diddling it or tossing it or bouncing it or teasing his neighbor with it—our task will be to begin to feel what we are doing.

First, then, we shall wait to feel what we have in our hands and not rush to do something with it. We shall take time to sense our relation to it. In a group there will be great individual differences in relation to the ball. There will be young fellows who have been playing baseball or basketball the day before and who, through long habituation, are more swiftly and fully focused by a ball than by anything else they touch; they are galvanized the moment a ball comes near them. And there will be others for whom old obligations to play ball have brought frustration and defeat. Then there are many who simply haven't had a ball in their hands for years.

So to begin with, we will all try to come to quiet. Let us specifically take time to allow more quiet in the region of our eyes: for many of us, just to have a ball in the hand means to be on the watch. Then we may sense our breathing. Here, too, we may clearly feel excitement, and any changes of the excitement toward calm. We take a reasonable time, letting it be or change as it will.

We will all try to come to quiet.

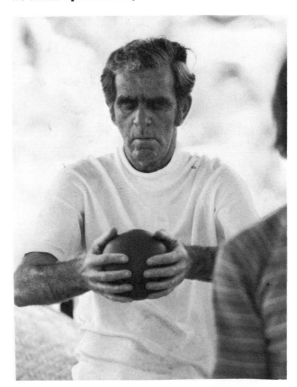

In any case, we now start to bounce the ball. How does it bounce? The reaction of the ball to the floor is a function of our own energy. We can bounce it higher or lower. Some of us have so much pent-up energy that it is hard to forgo this chance to let it out: our balls fly high. Very good. But what about breathing? Could some of the suppressed energy be allowed out in that? Not forced: *allowed*. Do we perhaps hold our breath to force out energy to bounce the ball? . . . Let us now not bounce the ball without at the same time sensing breathing.

We may give some time to let breathing gradually become freer as we bounce the ball. We may work to let our lips and brows become freer too. Many of us frown and purse our lips with each effort. Need it be an effort? Is there perhaps energy which could arise all by itself from our depths, as does a deep inhalation, without being caught and held in our expressions?

But bouncing a ball is not just throwing it at the floor. It is also receiving it as it returns. Here is perhaps a still more interesting study. If we were to pick out individuals from a group, many would show more anxiety in receiving the ball than in throwing it. Often we grab and clutch the ball as it bounces back to us, letting it take us off balance, suddenly becoming rigid all over as our arms stretch out for it and our hands close on it.

We have to go slowly as we begin to study receiving the ball. To clarify this a little we may now begin tossing the ball into the air. This requires somewhat more precision—in what I

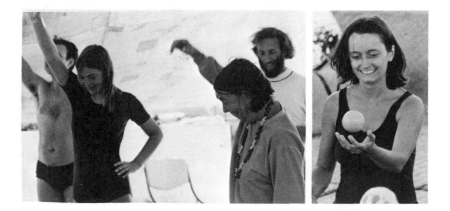

might now call the *giving* of the ball to space—than the bouncing did. Everyone is looking up now; there are apt to be collisions. One must toss the ball with a sense of direction, more or less straight up. What can we sense after tossing it? Do our hands and arms remain outstretched, stiff, anxiously awaiting the ball's return? If so, the ball will often simply bounce out of our rigid hands. We act as though receiving and giving were separate. Though we focus now on the moment of receiving the ball, in that moment we must also give to it.

It is not hard to get the idea of giving to the ball. Many people begin receiving the ball with bending arms, bending back, even deeply bending knees. It seems a little ostentatious. Indeed, it is not giving *to the ball*; it is one's *idea of giving*. Perhaps it is for the benefit of the group, perhaps for that of an unconscious inner audience. In any case, it represents a mental image of the "correct" way to do it. It is not functional.

Yet it is a beginning. We shall at least not become atrophied when we exaggerate. And it may be easily helped. When Charlotte, for instance, mimics such exaggerations before a group, the lesson is brought home immediately. A more difficult case, indeed, arises with experts, who also like to embellish their movements. An expert can be deeply involved in performing. With him, the embellishments may be very graceful and subtle, but this is still not *giving to the ball*. This can be a slippery and difficult question to work with. But such difficult questions are sometimes the most interesting and rewarding. This may be the time to add a new dimension to our study. Instead of merely giving the ball to space and receiving it as it returns, we may turn to giving and receiving, by means of the ball, with each other.[1]

A ball is the go-between *par excellence*, a messenger conveying a statement of attitude from one person to another. This attitude may be cooperative, competitive, hostile, friendly, exploratory—or any blend of these. It may also be lively or

---

1. Some of the fascinating range of the word *give*, with its inner positive and negative polarities—from the ferocious "Give it to him!" of a prizefight to opposite variations *give away, give in, give up*—becomes apparent here.

dull, deeply felt or shallowly. However it is, it can be illuminating to make a study of it.

For this purpose, let us divide the group into two halves, lined up opposite each other along two walls of the room. There is one ball for each pair; and the two simply toss it back and forth. Presently one group moves one place over, so that everybody has a new partner. These two play together for a while; then all change again, continuing this way until all partners have had perhaps half a dozen changes.

We will inquire now what anyone may have noticed. Were there differences between the different partners' ways of throwing and catching? Probably all were so involved in the demands of the play itself that they noticed very little. Sometimes the ball was harder to catch, sometimes easier. Once in a while, of course, there was an accident. That was all.

Let us continue, but this time with only half the group. The other half retires to one end of the room to watch, while those selected distribute themselves more amply this time along the two walls. Again the balls fly back and forth. They have quite different trajectories, some high, some low, some slow, some fast. We stop: one side moves over one place. We begin again, and so on.

By now several of the watchers have noticed that the fast balls tend to be thrown by the same persons, regardless of the partner. The fancy catches likewise tend to be made by the same persons, regardless of how the ball comes to them. This is not a simple, functional exchange. There is something extra in it.

The onlookers make their reports and then line up opposite each other to play in their turn. No matter what they may have noticed and reported about the first group, all this is apt to be forgotten when they come into action themselves. Such idiosyncrasies do not come from carelessness or ignorance, but from deeply ingrained personality traits. But at least as far as others are concerned, the group may already be becoming more discerning. It is not just fast balls and fancy catches that stand out. Certain persons, as before, will be seen to frown with every catch or press their lips with every throw. Others seem always startled or excessively cautious. The peculiarities become more complex.

We can try another approach. The whole group now returns to the two walls, facing each other. This time, before we start, each thrower takes care to see his partner—not looking at his eyes or his expression, not looking critically or with calculation, but yet seeing him fully. Then he tosses his ball *to that person.* The receiver is asked to let himself be more open and more there for the ball he receives. It goes slower now. With such a new orientation there may be many slips; that doesn't matter. We are eliminating what is competitive and habitual and beginning to play ball cooperatively.

As the pairs change to new pairs, this cooperation may well express itself in some cases with throws inviting a welcome reaching out by the receiver which for another receiver would be asking too much. Such possibilities are readily discovered and joyfully exploited. They are what gives the fun to playing and what gives the chance to each player to respond more vividly.

But let us see if a fuller cooperation is also possible in the simplest and easiest give and take—if we can be as awake and present when the ball is simply handed to us. The two groups are now asked, as they continue tossing the balls back and forth, to come closer to each other. Throws that would make extra demands on the other would now be extravagant. As the members of each pair approach each other, with ever-shortening tosses they become more and more awake for the ball and for the other. The time comes when no more space is left. The ball must pass directly from hand to hand. We go very slowly and finally pause. The presence of each can be felt, through the ball, by the other. We start backward toward the walls, continuing to toss—but in our tissues we now know something of who it is we toss to.

We shall work again, though perhaps not in this same class, with exchanging balls. But this time we will not bounce or toss or throw them. We will simply approach another person and give our ball to him, and feel how we receive it when a ball is given to us. We have already done this with the more beautiful and interesting stones. But when we have allowed time enough for preparation, this act of giving whatever is in our hands to the hands of another can become a true act of giving, one in which the intrinsic value of the object given means less than the sharing of a common humanity. Caring, seriousness, and joy show in the faces of people so engaged.[1]

One of Charlotte's favorite ways of ending a workshop is to let each participant stand by his ball as it rests on the floor. He then nudges it with his foot, and as it rolls he follows it as if he were its shadow, to right or left, fast or slow, through the thick of things till finally both ball and person slow down, perhaps wobble a little, and at last come to rest.

Nothing could require more attention than this. One's response must be immediate, instantaneous. At first it seems impossible to lessen the gap between what one does to the ball and how one follows it. One is asked to supply energy as one throws a switch. Yet there is no magic in it: every bird in a flock, every fish in a school moves this way. Every skier must respond in this way to the changes in the slope. As we are neither in danger nor in competition, there is nothing special to achieve. When we fail to follow the ball, it doesn't matter. But when we begin to feel what is asked of us, we may have a revelation.

1. See Appendix C.

33 SENSING ONE'S OWN HEAD

The essence of sensory awareness lies in distinguishing our actual experience from our thoughts and fantasies. Yet it is rather with the latter that we have generally come to identify ourselves. We like to think of intellectual processes as bringing us nearer to a cosmic order and harmony than is the case with our fellow creatures. This presumption, I suppose, must remain forever questionable. For what Blake saw in the eye that dared frame the tiger (which perhaps was the tiger's eye itself), and what we may see in every alerted eye that beholds us from the zoo,[1] may be the very wonder we feel also when consciousness plays freely among all the organs and tissues of our head, and is not restricted to reasoning.

Nevertheless, though we all agree in desiring keen senses, and take much satisfaction in clear vision and acute hearing and sensitive love-making, this is as nothing to the importance we attach to clear and keen thinking and to the admiration we feel for it, either in ourselves or in others. "Reason," we are convinced, and perhaps rightly, is the crowning glory of man.

But how we arrive at reason is another matter. We have been taught that clear thinking depends on concentration, or the act of shutting out irrelevancies, and that concentration, in turn, depends upon an act of will. Since childhood, we have been urged to pay attention and to *think*. Obediently imitating our teachers, we frown and purse our lips when confronting a problem in arithmetic or morals, just as we did when tossing and catching balls. Tightened jaws and contorted brows follow —indeed anything forceful to give us the feeling we are in

1. Cf. note page 109.

control of things and are confining ourselves to problem-solving. But unfortunately, all this does not do what it is supposed to; it only distorts our perception and helps make thinking rigid and compulsive. This is why it is shocking to compare the efforts so often visible in the face of a schoolchild doing his homework with the tranquillity that could be seen in his face a few years earlier and that can still be seen in the portraits of Einstein and Shakespeare.

It is not our concern here that "geniuses" follow deep natural interests, while the schoolchild may be occupied with the very opposite. We are not concerned with a critique of education, but only with our reactions to the educational, methods of prodding and insisting to which, through no fault of our own, we were all exposed.

The trouble is that we have been led into creating a problem where none exists. As a cat is totally alerted, and its attention focused, by the appearance of a mouse, so our minds focus entirely by themselves when a real occasion presents itself. It is just our fantasy that one must "grasp" an idea as one grasps a stick, or "cudgel our brains" to make them work. But this is what has happened to us; and it is to unveil for ourselves some of the consequent incessant activities going on just under our scalps and façades that in our classes we sometimes work on sensing our own heads.

■ Standing or sitting, we may close our eyes and let our head come to more resting on the tissues below it.

We may be asked, as Elsa Gindler used to ask, "Do you feel anything where you suppose your head is?"

Sensations are apt to be very vague. We are allowed ample time.

"Can you feel anything in the space between your ears?" . . . More time . . . "Between your temples?"

To one seeing a group in this situation, their expressions are striking. The mask of daily living is already fading, an unwonted attentiveness and quiet spreading over each figure.

"Can you feel the distance between your eyes? . . . Do you allow the room needed for whatever exists there?"

In the time allowed for sensing the region between the eyes, a whole microcosm may begin to stir into consciousness. Very slowly we proceed.

"Can you feel anything of what exists between your cheeks? . . . Of where the air enters?" . . . Much time . . . "Of the space across your jaws?" . . . "Can you feel the roof of your mouth?"

Every facial expression with which we have learned to greet and confront the world, or to mask ourselves from it, has its roots below the surface. Now that our attention has been led to the soil where these roots intermingle, astonishing connections begin to reveal themselves. A tangle of deep-lying muscles may stir, shift, give way, as the various features and organs we were born with begin striving, after years of conditioning, to find their natural places and relationships. From our faces deep inner releases are draining the characteristics by which others know us. One seeing us now might find many of us blank, our features as yet unable to fill out the elusive freedom they dimly begin to sense. This will take long practice. Yet in us altogether is an atmosphere of growing inner awakeness and presence. Consciousness has not been lessened but rather heightened; it has only been turned inward.

We may now be asked to open our eyes and look around. For a moment, the scene is like a fresh morning, with dew on every flower.

In reporting experiences, many people will have discovered tensions around eyes, nostrils, et cetera, which began to dissolve by themselves when attention was maintained and time allowed. Some will have noticed accompanying changes in breathing and greater freedom in standing or sitting, as the case may have been. Also the muscles of the scalp may have become conscious here and there, giving some sense of dimension and of the mass in the interior (occasionally giving up the contractions that had been causing a headache); while everywhere in the head interweavings of muscle tissue and organic function were felt to some degree. Constrictions around eyes, ears, nose, and throat, and everywhere in between, becoming conscious, became also to some extent relieved.

A fascinating element in this sensing of the inner head is

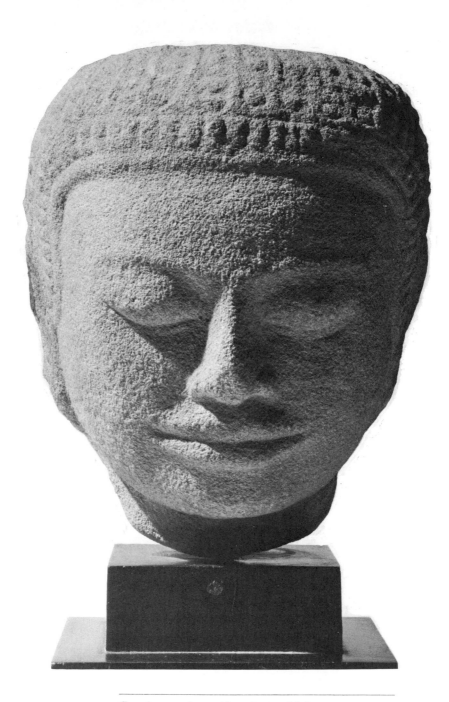

**Consciousness has not been lessened but,
rather, heightened.**

the common recognition that the head consists of the same living tissues as the rest of the organism. In fact, in complexity at least, it may be felt to be our most densely muscular region and may, indeed, be that region where the greatest variety of voluntary muscles habitually works involuntarily. These involuntary workings, or reflexes—our characteristic facial expressions—tend, with our characteristic ways of speaking, to identify us to other people. They affect our sensations, our attitudes, our thoughts, which can literally be felt changing and coming to a new life precisely as the muscular basis of these expressions begins to become conscious.

When the proprioceptive sensory nerves are awakened, so that the eyes, ears, and nostrils for once become the objects of sensation and not, as usually, just sensors, consciousness begins to flow as naturally throughout the organism as the circulating blood. As inhibitions relent in the musculature of these organs, and their vigilance ebbs, releases may be felt in all the related muscular systems everywhere. No longer is it head and body, no longer mind and body.[2] This mind is not the function of the computing brain, nor is it at home only in the brain's neighborhood, near the special senses that orient us and give us our everyday perspective on the world. It is a function of the organism altogether. The ten billion cells of the brain, occupying that great area inside our head where we can feel nothing, can be only its infinitely complicated switchboard.

2. See Introduction pages 8–10.

34 TOWARD
EXPANDED CONSCIOUSNESS

Elsa Gindler's first name for what Charlotte Selver later called "sensory awareness" was *Nachentfaltung*—the "unfolding afterward." Frequently, the after effects of classes are the most significant. During my first years with Charlotte in New York, when I worked during the day and attended classes in the evening, I would often walk afterward for half an hour or so down the dark streets, savoring the quiet exhilaration of just being alive. I could feel with joy my own movements in walking and the ceaseless activity of my own breathing. Great dark office buildings lined the almost empty avenues north of Times Square; against the background of their walls and the unbroken pavement, I sensed the aliveness of the few figures passing me.

Once in a while at night, and sometimes even more among the crowded streets by day, it would come to me that all these people, no matter how unconscious of it, shared with me the great fact of being alive at this moment. Each, like me, was a bud that had formed this year on the tree of life, unfolding and growing in his own way before dying, no matter how conditioned by circumstances. In this light, each of us seemed to have a preciousness beyond all good and evil, and beyond anything that one of us could do to the other. At these moments, something in me bowed invisibly to each passer-by.

Years later, a weekend of very concentrated work brought a somewhat similar heightening of consciousness. This time I happened to be the leader. The experience lasted six hours or more, and I could and did avail myself of an opportunity for recording it. I offer it here approximately as it was noted down at the time.

■   In April 1971 I was invited by the only psychiatrist in a southern Idaho town to give a weekend workshop in the population center of this farming country, which had once been a sagebrush desert traversed by the Snake River. All the participants were local. It was raining on my arrival Friday afternoon and still raining when I left on Sunday—a very unusual event for this arid land. During the weekend, I took a few short walks on the farm road among the large and—at this season—rather characterless fields, getting a little fresh air mixed with snow flurries and rain. Otherwise my attention was entirely given to the workshop, my hosts, and my own periods of resting.

The work with this relatively unfamiliar group of professional people and their wives, from a generally conservative farming region, did not go as clearly and compellingly as I should have wished; and on Sunday morning I felt a great need to get something across in the short time still available. We worked with the feel of a stone resting in our hands, and then with coming freely to sitting on the folding chairs. At the end of this experiment, one sat while another touched his chest and diaphragm, feeling what could be sensed of living process within, for which room might be better allowed in sitting.

We lay down briefly to rest, and came up to standing. It seemed that everyone could still feel his existence where the other's hands had come to him, and could feel the possibility in standing of allowing life there. A circle formed by itself, and we held hands in farewell. Everyone seemed moved, as I was also.

The departure of the only plane back left no time for lingering. I packed, had a little lunch, and was driven to the airport in the slightly exalted state I feel when conscious of acting swiftly, but unhurriedly and economically.

All went on schedule, and I was soon airborne.

■   *Twin Falls–Boise, 2 p.m.* Overcast and rain, high enough to permit view of country, but not full sense of distance. Hoping to see the Sawtooth Mountains, I was able to take a starboard seat. As we took off and gained altitude, the farmlands lay plainly to be seen: each different field, and each house and yard in its space among the fields—the house sheltered more or less with trees, so that the feeling of what was there for *living*, in relation to the house, was so clearly different from what was there for *earning* a living. Here, they had told me, all had been sagebrush and desert; now it was all either for each man's personal enjoyment, or for his wealth and society's loss or gain (losing the beauty of the desert, or gaining potatoes and alfalfa, however one might see it).

No mountains came into sight as we climbed: only the gathering denseness of the clouds we now began to enter. Then through the mist I saw the Snake River canyon, a long gash worn deep into the plain. As I looked, it dimmed and disappeared, and I was left with undifferentiated gray light outside the window. Inside was the clear and unchanged (but now isolated and unrelated) interior of the plane, to which the visible world of form was now reduced.

Would I still see the mountains, which I had not seen since my arrival forty-eight hours ago? Or was reality what I saw and felt now, so much reduced as it was? Without effort, I felt inner changes leading consciousness away from imagination, away from thought, to my own breathing. A need to leave the contoured back of the seat led me from it into a gentle stretching of back and pelvis and into the more independent sitting toward which we had been working in the workshop that morning. I loosened the seat belt. More and more, consciousness grew to include the felt with the seen—the latter still present, though so much of it was only a uniform gray light. Could it be that this was *it*, as I had asked the group about the stone to which each one was invited to give his attention a few hours earlier? The words of Suzuki-roshi came to me: "Zazen sitting *is* Enlightenment." More and more I felt the gentle pleasure of existing, free of the seat back, in my back and pelvis, the pleasure of sensitive, unplanned movements in spine and organs, the pleasure of the gentle movement of breathing.

I was sitting relatively upright in the plane, and I realized that I had never sat so in a plane before. There was another passenger in the aisle seat of my row, but I sensed that I was in no way blocking his view or even intruding on his awareness. It did not seem that my unusual posture was noticed by anyone in the plane. But it was now not important that it was "unusual"; it was merely conscious and delicious.

In the background of consciousness hovered the recognition that "Enlightenment" might be no mental or verbalizable process of any sort, but mere "physical" sensation. I felt a delightful absence of heaviness: it was as though it was light in me (in either sense of the word), while outside of me all was light in its two aspects: pure and without form out the window, only forms in the interior.

The cloud was thinning now, and we emerged above it, my eyes filling with lovely soft forms, whitish and grayish, spreading out beneath clear space, traced with vapors still well above us. Higher still, the clear speck of a long-distance jet plane appeared and was lost. Then we nosed gently back into the cloud. I pulled out my watch: we were just over half way, fifteen minutes from take-off. We would not climb higher, even if the mountains were high enough to be visible above the overcast.

Again all was forms in the plane's interior, light without form out the window, and the living me. Still I felt the pleasure of inner movements in sitting, free of the back of the seat, as the recognition came that this is why one *sits* in meditation, instead of leaning or lying.

The plane was sinking. Now we were emerging beneath the clouds. A new landscape appeared, houses less cozily planned, it seemed to me; a big town to the north; not far away, snow-capped mountains. A few giants appeared dimly in the distance. Really, they were not so interesting: it was more my idea about them than the visual experience that had affected me.

Perhaps something else out ahead was far more real—if so, a reality fast approaching. *I might be killed in the landing.* Fear gripped me, slowing my breath, which I then deliberately permitted. But as I permitted breathing, the sharpness of my recognition slipped away.

I tried to get it back. Could I accept imminent death as a real possibility? It came to me strongly that "full enlightenment" would include a full acceptance of this possibility, which I could feel so much of me pushing back into the world of the intellect. Could I accept *it*—the present with a clear possibility of death in a moment? What was death? It involved others, who perhaps needed me. But *it* would be a now, including "death," without qualification. Dimly I sensed the inner readjustments that might constitute such acceptance: readjustments that seemed more "physical" than "mental," if I were to use such words. Now the moment was at hand. I tried to realize that *it really might happen now*. All my knowledge told me this was so: could all my organism admit this contribution of "mind," as the blood stream admits the contribution of the stomach? I shivered; but it was already too late to tell. My division into mind and body was still too strong. We were touching down— we *had* touched down: the odds against catastrophe were too great. It could only be imagination now. The chance was lost. Forget it! The now, for better or worse, had left behind this particular chance for accepting the whole, if indeed it had ever been a chance.

Now the reality was that I could put some of the experience into words, if I would take the trouble. There was a two-hour wait—time enough. As I entered the airport building, I saw the waiting room entirely empty. I chose a seat in the far corner and took out paper and pen.

■   When I reached San Francisco, there was an even longer wait for the short flight to Monterey.

Notes written in San Francisco airport, 8:30 p.m. At six p.m., the limousine into the city. I walk through empty Sunday streets toward Chinatown. The green grass and palms of Union Square a background for blazing colors of rhododendrons and primroses. A few stragglers from the peace march. Along Grant Avenue to the Yee Jun.

At a tiny table, I order seaweed soup and asparagus beef. On a column beside me hangs a mirror; glancing, I see my own face and eyes. They are real and content me.

A great bowl of seaweed soup is set before me, steaming in

the chill that flows down the open stairway from the street. I realize I should not have ordered anything else, but it is too late. I begin. The soup's heat and its ingredients enter my mouth. My eyes, though lowered, feel powerfully open. A roaring energy of the restaurant, the sounds and movements of closely packed, hungry, eating people, seems to come to me through ears, eyes, and all my pores. Equivalent to this energy from the environment, my own inner energy becomes conscious: a power in my own breathing which carries me along with it; a giant in me stirring, overpowering habitual resistances in me with no sense of effort.

There is hardly room in me for eating, despite my empty stomach. I eat notwithstanding: the hot broth, the mass of seaweed, tough bits of gizzard—but without my usual ravenousness. Habit urges me to gobble, but breathing and awareness are now so much stronger that to follow my habit would be a violence against myself. The hands of the clock turn: my time for the return limousine is running out. I will not be able to look for a Chinese gong. But perhaps only one errand is important—the oranges from the stand at Stockton and Jackson. If I catch the Stockton Street bus to the limousine terminal, there is time for that. It is wonderful how my overwhelming new awarenesses leave room for awareness of all practical necessities. These are not dimmed but very clear.

To limousine, ten minutes early, with oranges. Seated before me on the right, two homosexuals, one newly barbered, with sallow flesh in face and throat, the other ruddy. On the left, the loud aggressiveness of two square heterosexuals. A pale, quiet figure sits beside me. There is no tension between its hormones and mine. My bag of oranges tips on the floor, and one orange rolls against its feet. I turn to excuse myself as I reach down for the orange. It is a young woman. She has a Mexican bag, like mine. Should I speak to her? There is no need for it. No sense of aggressiveness from or toward her, positive or negative. Beneath her quiet, perhaps her colorlessness, I sense a living being and feel its validity, even its perfectness.

Again I realize I am in a far higher state of awareness than usual. Out the limousine window, I see trees bowing before the wind and a dense fog bank creeping down over the San Bruno hills. But I realize I only see them and do not experience them: I am becoming the reporter.

In the airport, I get my bag of stones from the locker, add the bag of oranges, and sit waiting for the Monterey plane. Before me is a sickly woman, berating two sickly little children in straw hats, with toy guns and flags. They move away. A young man and woman sit where they were. The young man's hand grabs and drums on the woman's sides and back. Irritation at his insensitivity disturbs me, but evidently not the woman. On the contrary, she leans closer to him. Seeing them now together, I feel what she feels of his desire for her through his roughness. My irritation leaves. My eyes are on them; they realize this, but are not disturbed. My sense of their sense of each other becomes stronger, overpowering. They get up and move to seats a little less in the center of things, and I can feel the genuineness and simplicity of the contact which I can no longer see.

On the plane from San Francisco to Monterey I make these last notes. The plane is late for its brief flight; it is already almost dark. As I glance out the window westward, there is an extraordinary sight: a rim, as of rosé wine, to the horizon, and set in it the least sliver of a moon. Between it and the plane billows the same pure sea of clouds I had seen over Idaho, but now many shades away from white and nearer black. But as with the wind and fog outside the limousine, I know, as I do not usually know, that I cannot now experience it, even though I find fitting words. I am writing, and my cup is already full.

As I hurry to get these last notes on paper, the stewardess announces our descent to Monterey, and I must snap on my seat belt.

35 SENSORY AWARENESS IN COMMUNICATION

Heightened consciousness arising from meditation is an end in itself. Don Juan, in the books of Castaneda, simply *saw*.[1] But there are others who see (including Castaneda himself) who need to communicate. For them a medium is necessary, in which they can find some equivalent to their perception.

Words, the prime medium of man, which we all learn as children, may tell our story. Oftener, they lead us away from it.

Color, line, and sound are surer. But, using these, we are on the open sea. We cannot look up a color or a tone in the dictionary. So art and music schools work hard to create such dictionaries, studying and pinning down the "techniques" of great painters and composers, and setting up authorities, while others who also seek to show the way petrify the experience of their authorities in symbols.

But no one's experience can be found in a dictionary, or in a cross or a mandala.

Thus Suzuki-roshi entitled his book *Zen Mind, Beginner's Mind*,[2] and starts out, "In the beginner's mind there are many possibilities, but in the expert's there are few."

During the last half-century, communication has become the subject of widespread study. It is no longer taken for granted, as was true formerly. Psychologists, philosophers, and artists have pushed off from terra firma into unknown seas. In this book, various means have been explored to study the phenom-

1. Op. cit. See pages 5–6.

2. Shunryu Suzuki, *Zen Mind, Beginner's Mind* (New York: Weatherhill, 1971).

ena of perceiving and relating, the twin functions from which communication arises.

■ Now, in conclusion, I should simply like to offer an example. I wish to set down now a few recollections of the artist and the man who, of all men, made the greatest impression on my life; who affected my earlier years as Charlotte Selver affected my maturity. He approached his canvases as she approaches her classes. In his mind, as in hers, as he began a work, I believe everything was possible, for it was all new. This man was the American painter Arthur Dove.

In our studio in New York, one small painting hangs on the wall. It depicts a single hollyhock. There may be a few branches and flowers in the room, there is a much-loved weaving, and on the floor is a heap of stones from the beach in Maine. But nothing has the intense individuality of the *Hollyhock*, or glows with the life and movement of its few lines and colors.

I was in the same room with Arthur Dove in the summer of 1935 when something impelled him to begin the single black line on a piece of paper which grew in zigzag, curling, dropping, climbing to its completion. The hand that drew followed some deep inner rhythm, pausing here and there in its course to sense a moment before looping off. There was no haste, no hesitation. Then a brush dipped briefly in watercolor, a calm, sensuous spreading of red and green, and it was over.

The next year when I bought the *Hollyhock* from Stieglitz's gallery, I could only write Dove that it gave me a sensation of joy and quick movement in my insides. It was like the kick of a baby in the womb or a calypso dance.

It was in the early twenties, when Dove was trying to make ends meet by raising chickens and catching lobsters in Connecticut, that his son and I became bosom friends. Few real experiences were shared by the men and boys of the community, and it was a vivid interlude when Dove took three of us camping. There was no fuss or formality. We just took what we needed and walked a mile and a half out of town to the wilderness of an abandoned millpond. For us twelve-year-olds, a quarter-mile of our own still contained the world. We had our

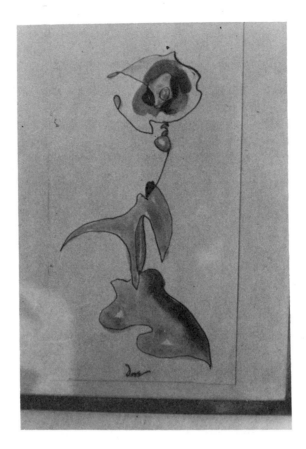

tent, our fire, our food, and no adult programing. Dove was just present in his way as the woods were in theirs, and his presence gave a cohesiveness and depth to the experience which it would have lacked without him.

I have no other memories of Dove at that time. He soon separated from his wife, remarried, and moved to Long Island. But about 1930, I began to go on Christmas vacations with his son to visit him. We went for perhaps three visits of a day or two each to the teetering old "yacht club" on a harbor in the Sound, where he lived rent-free with his wife, Reds, in exchange for keeping the rowboats tied up during winter storms. Inside, a coal stove glowed against the draughts and rattles, while Arthur and Reds seemed to me like the glow of life itself. We boys brought cheese and bootleg wine which we picked up on our way through New York, Reds had a steaming stew, and Arthur produced his homemade gin. When we were full and had talked a while over the wine, we wrapped up in all available covers and slept.

The next morning after breakfast, in that bright winter sunlight, with snow on the deck and the gulls soaring and wheeling just out the windows, Arthur would bring out his year's work. They were oil paintings, not very big, with brilliant, uncompromising colors and strange forms that baffled and somehow frightened me. This was not the world I had spent my twenty years learning and coming to terms with, but something very different that I could not explain to myself or understand. Nor was Arthur any help. Once he explained to his great friend, the painter Alfie Maurer, who had come out on the train with us, that some painting was " like holding an egg in your hand." Though these words have stayed in my mind for forty years, at the time he might as well have spoken in Chinese. So I looked and looked and said nothing, and felt great relief when the paintings were put away and we could just go back to being such warm human beings together.

Soon afterward, Dove inherited a tumbledown old farmhouse in upstate New York. It had an outdoor privy and a pump outside the kitchen door for water. One winter morning, on a visit there, when I tried to pour the water from my bedroom pitcher into the bowl, I found it frozen solid. To my young urban eyes this was quite romantic. It was long before I realized how much the Doves were both paying in privation and effort for the privilege of living close to nature and working as they chose.

Then one evening by the coal stove we had a talk on art. I said that for me there was one painter, Rembrandt; and Dove said there was something else. I had in mind the engravings of the Crucifixion, and I spoke of what seemed to me, an atheist, the overwhelmingly wonderful religious feelings of Rembrandt and his depiction of man's relation to the Unknown. Dove maintained that art had another function, but what it was he was perfectly unable to make clear to me. He was not a naturally verbal person, and I must have assaulted him with theories and interpretations. In any case, the effort was too much for him, and about nine-thirty—an hour past his normal bedtime—he fell asleep.

In the morning, after breakfast, I felt very quiet. The others, including Arthur, had things to do, and when I found myself alone I went straight to the little upstairs bedroom which was his studio. There was no furniture, the walls were bare and white, and a pure north light came in through the shaky windows. Here, in a world of their own, hung this year's paintings, blood brothers of all the others that had so confused me before. The colors were strong and brilliant, the forms strange. I stopped before one a little less remote to me than the others: it was clearly the morning sun over a ploughed field, with what must be trees or shrubbery in the background. I had seen one somewhat like it by Van Gogh. But Van Gogh's distortions I recognized as power of emotion, as struggle, love, rage, apocalypse. Here I could find no clue for interpretation—only something that held me. Then in the center of the sun itself a black splotch caught my eye; and as I began to look at this splotch and wonder why it was there, I began to feel sunburned. Nothing like this had ever happened to me. I could feel the sun burning me from the canvas. Furthermore, there was a feeling as though I were standing in a shower with streams coming down on me. Streams of something—perhaps sunbeams or the rays of the plowed field. My questioning vanished, leaving me with a sense of quiet and exhilaration. Here was something that could simply be felt. It did not need to be understood.

Across the little room, I now noticed something quite different but equally easy to see. It was a sun setting behind clouds on a calm evening. The clouds, in gentle hues, were silhouetted over one another, line beyond line, and as my eye ran along their edges I felt the living lines, just as I had felt the living linear movement in Bach's Brandenburg Concertos. And just as I had listened to these merely with delight, and without the need for "understanding," this was now possible for me for the first time before a painting.

Still another painting now caught my attention. This was more difficult. Unlike the others, it was flat areas of color, no gradations or nuances, just bald statements. Across the colors rose the jagged form of a black iron bridge. The day before, I could not have endured to look at anything so stark and toneless. This seemed an aggressive wasteland. And then before my eyes it began to move, in great rhythms rising and crashing like a Beethoven symphony—a totality of rhythm with which I could only live for a few moments.

I left the room and walked for a little by myself. These paintings were the very substance of the man I loved to be near. They were not something he could explain, but something he had experienced and cherished and given on. They were no philosophy, no religion, no scenes from nature: they just *were*.

When I saw him, I asked if what he had painted was the Bach and the Beethoven. I didn't use these names, but tried to express the quality of movement by gestures. A joy of recognition flowed between us. The door had opened for me.

Later I tried to play Beethoven records to him, but they bored him. All he liked in music was Louis Armstrong and ragtime.[3] And when I read him the chapter in *Moby Dick* on the Whiteness of the Whale, which for me had something of the same wonder he had himself, he fell asleep. Perhaps to be really oneself in the 1930s was a full-time task that could admit no historical influences. And, except for one or two Zen roshis, Dove seems to me almost the only man I have ever known, at least in the United States, who was really himself.

In the evening he showed me paintings from other years. I had entered their world, and wherever my gaze fell was living form and color. Strange shapes and figures greeted me with the movements of my own experience, with the tones of my own feelings, enlarged and affirmed. These were no fantasies, no symbols; they were representations of the real world as Dove had experienced it, and as I experienced it through him. Thirty

3. Stieglitz's favorite Dove was probably *Louis Armstrong: Swing Music*, now in the Art Institute, Chicago. When I worked in 1962 with Charlotte's teacher Heinrich Jacoby, in Zurich, the only thing he asked me about the United States was, "Were there any other Louis Armstrongs?" It seemed recordings were hard to get in Switzerland.

years later, I would have similar experiences through our own classes, and once or twice under LSD. They stilled my thoughts and directly aroused my perception as no art ever had before.

In the few years that followed when I was in or near New York, I never missed a Dove show at An American Place. As nearly as possible, Alfred Stieglitz let things speak for themselves. It was a gallery of utter simplicity, a few blocks across from the fashionable Museum of Modern Art. Few people came, and there were several small, bare, white rooms where one could be alone with a painting until one had come to the quiet of mind that would permit it to speak. These paintings were certainly nothing one could take in at a glance. Nor were they even anything one could study, or interpret or compare critically, as I in my first experience had with composers. One could only be alone with a painting, and when the commotion one had brought along with one had died down, it would begin to *be*.

In the summer of 1935, the summer of the *Hollyhock*, I again visited the farmhouse and found Arthur and Reds full of excitement about a new painting. Have you ever seen *Farrebique*, the film of a year's changes on a French farm? Later it was skillfully imitated by Disney in his *Living Desert*. Through an adroit use of the camera, plants grow, buds swell and open as you watch. It was very sensitively made and is thrilling to see. But *Farrebique* was about 1950, and the time I am speaking of was long before.

There was a conspiratorial tone in the Doves' voices as they spoke of *The Goat*, and as soon as I found myself alone I went upstairs to see it. A small painting, as I realized many years later when I saw it again, but that afternoon it looked like the whole wall of the room. In fact, there was space in it for a snowy mountain range, at one end of which floated sleeping a full moon—only really it was a goat's head, eyes closed, and the mountain range was the brown and white outline of his back, silently undulating from head to tail, where my eye plunged down the thigh and leg and came upon a chasm, above which a great, curving, brownish shape grew, filling the picture. I caught my breath as I saw it was the goat's erection, or rather the whole goat becoming erection, growing and swelling toward a vast cleft, warm and deep as the night or as the earth itself. Ebbing from the closed eyes and brain of the moonlike head, life flowed along the gleaming heights of the back, and down, down through earthy loins into an infinitely sensitive growing edge that hovered above an equally sensitive unfolding.

What a masterly cinematographer did later with the life in plants, Dove had done here in motionless oil on canvas with the ultimate relationship possible in all animal life.

This is the only painting I have ever seen, from any period, in which the act of love is not in any way illustrated or symbolized, but is fully felt through and reproduced in materials. As Stieglitz called his photographs, this is truly an *equivalent*.

I find it fascinating that so much of the organismic and orgastic trend in the avant-garde philosophies, poetry, and psychotherapies of the last two or three decades should have been fully anticipated in the deeply grounded and unrelenting connection which, in his isolation, Dove established with natural process.

Dove died long before anyone in my world had ever heard of Zen. But I would not hesitate to describe him as a Zen master. I believe that, whatever his intellectual development, in his long maturity he painted in quiet, practically without theory and with full attention. And there was nothing in the world of nature from which he shrank. He and Reds were a full world in themselves; they lived secluded and in the humblest way, seeing hardly anyone. But at the Ketewomoke Yacht Club, where every rowboat owner was Captain Jones or Captain Smith, it was once said to him—the overseer of the fleet—"I like to go yachting with you, Commodore!"

For with Dove people came into more connection with the reality of the water beneath and of the wind around and of the little rowboat in the midst of it. Not through anything he said; simply through his presence, as it had been with us twelve-year-olds in the woods. This was not just a visual or imaginary connection, as with most people and most painters, but a connection of the total organism, as between the two elements in *The Goat*. That this connection could reach the canvas, and through that me and others, was possible only because between world and canvas was interposed no preconception and no calculation, but only the living pathways of a man.

The war came and went. After seven years away, I saw Arthur again in 1946, three months before his death. He and Reds were living where I had seen them last, in the little abandoned post office they had finally bought on the pond in Centerport, Long Island. They had raised the floors after being flooded in a hurricane, and they had insulated the walls so it was at last warm and cozy. For Reds, who had roughed it so long with her frail health and unflagging spirit, it was a home at last. But Arthur was bedridden. In order to paint as he had to in a world which had little interest in the message of the senses, he had never spared himself. He and Reds had accepted all the challenges and insecurities that had confronted them over many years and in many dwellings where disaster was often about to strike. At last, for him everything had given in together—lungs, heart, and kidneys. They had made new friends: the local doctor, who refused a fee, and a nurse from the state hospital who lovingly helped Reds to care for him. But the man who had always done everything for himself, from grinding his own colors to keeping his own habitations afloat or standing, could no longer walk across the room. And yet, immobilized, he was as much all there as when I had first met him, as fully present in the real world with which he never had lost touch, as most of us do. He still painted. One of the most moving of his paintings had been done while he was ill in bed. This was *Neighborly Attempt at Murder*,[4] and I doubt if any work of art ever sprang more directly from the soil of the present.

Into the house nearest the Doves had moved an unhappy family. Often there was shouting at the two young children and quarrels between husband and wife. One night instead of shouts there were shrieks. For minutes and minutes, perhaps hours, there were shrieks, first of rage and then of terror. Later Reds learned that the woman had fought off the man and

4. Collection of William Lane Found., Leominster, Massachusetts.

succeeded in killing herself, and had almost succeeded in killing the two children.

Arthur had lain in bed, unable to move. The next day he was unable to speak. The second day he was still unable to speak. On the third day, Reds assembled paints and canvas for him, and he worked without a word until all was set down.

Neighborly Attempt at Murder is a combination of pure tone and movement. Unspeakable depths and relationships take form and color. Perhaps it is something like what Rembrandt might have done with the *Crucifixion*, had he been present on that occasion and had it been possible in that epoch for him to come to painting without preconceptions, with a lifetime of experience and work, but with a beginner's mind.

Epilogue

I n working together even for very short periods in sensory awareness, a group of people develop a sense of respect and affection for one another which is not often met with. For we are working on our common humanity, on those fundamental attributes which antedate our many divergent cultures. Though our groups seldom afford the drama (and melodrama) of "encounter groups," with their verbal confrontation, a very direct and deep meeting of people, in sensitivity and quiet emotional honesty, is possible, using no techniques, in the usual sense, at all. In the longer workshops, many of our students form good and friendly relations with the people in the community, no matter how conservative the community may be in other respects. For we are beginning to lose our *ideas about* our behavior, and beginning to feel how our behavior *is*. Though our work, in its nature, tends to subvert and undermine every institution, it is only to let in the fresh air and sunshine which institutions keep out. To the extent that he can accept the sunshine, everyone feels he becomes a little more human; and as he accepts a little, he becomes able to accept more. Finally he finds he can accept the city with the country, or the country with the city; and the night with the day.

As I have said, despite the immediate delights, the work is slow. Distraction alternates with perception, and resistance with insight. The attention flags; one tires. The road can seldom be direct, so we must be prepared for detours. In other words, our sessions are work and require discipline. But if the discipline is imposed by the leader, it will defeat its purpose. He must instead, by his own presence and experience (or, lacking that, by his skill) arouse the interest in the group which will guide their attention and tide them over the shallows.

We have, therefore, a difficult task, though a delightful one. We must seek the aliveness in ourselves which awakens it in others. If we instruct and explain, we do what has already been done in our usual education, even when it seems to contradict this education on the surface. We merely substitute a new authority for the old. If we play games, using techniques which we have found are sensational, we fall into another pit, where perhaps everyone has had fun, but little insight has been gained. Of the two sidetracks, the first may have an intellectual influence, with possibly some political or social value, while the second may shake people out of certain habits and entice them into new pleasures which may be felt as liberating. I myself have oscillated between these two sidetracks in years of teaching. But it is like that muddy water which often must be pumped from a well before the clear water flows. And the fact that the muddy water may be useful does not mean that one should not continue to seek the clear. When the clear water begins to come (and it may come, and disappear for long periods, and come again), it is unmistakable.

Such clear water, flowing everywhere among a group of people, may—as Charlotte says it is her only task to do—penetrate through their skin and stir them awake.

Appendices

A ELSA GINDLER:
ARBEIT AM MENSCHEN

The term "sensory awareness" has become widely used in recent years, often with little knowledge either of its significance or of its origin. It was first coined by Charlotte Selver, about 1950, as a name for her version of a work originated by Elsa Gindler in Berlin, some forty years earlier.

Gindler was a teacher of physical education, who fell ill of tuberculosis in her early twenties and was given up by the doctors, being left with the advice to quit the city and spend her remaining days in the pure air of the Alps. For a young teacher of working-class parents, this was out of the question.

There was then no technique of collapsing the diseased lung to allow it to rest. But Gindler had the intuition that with quiet and patience she might be able to sense something of her own inner processes and find ways to encourage healing rather than hinder it. The tissues involved being those of one side of her lungs, she felt it was her task to become so sensitive in breathing that she could allow breathing in the healthy side of her lungs only, while the seriously infected other side could remain relatively at rest.

This self-imposed task might almost be considered a definition of what Zen Buddhist students now call "meditation"— total involvement with breathing—although in 1910 Gindler had certainly never heard of Zen and was experimenting entirely on her own. Since breathing involves more of the large musculature than any other basic life activity, this meant an awakening to her own inner flexibilities and processes on a very general scale. Indeed, it meant an alerting of the entire sensory nervous system, for, like a pebble dropped in water, an excitation at any point in the organism tends to set up reactions everywhere. In so critical a situation, every disturbance in breathing was acute. On the other hand, when the inner functioning could be sensed, hindrances could consciously be allowed to dissolve and cease interfering with the organism's innate tendencies to regeneration.

This discovery and practice of Gindler's is the basis of our entire work.

In a year, Elsa Gindler had indeed healed herself, to the bafflement of her academic doctors, one of whom, meeting her by chance on the street and asking her to come to his office for an examination, turned red in the face at her explanation of the cure and exclaimed gruffly, "Wonders can sometimes happen!"

But from then on she felt unable to continue teaching calisthenics. She was fired with the recognition that to learn to

---

Elsa Gindler, 1945.

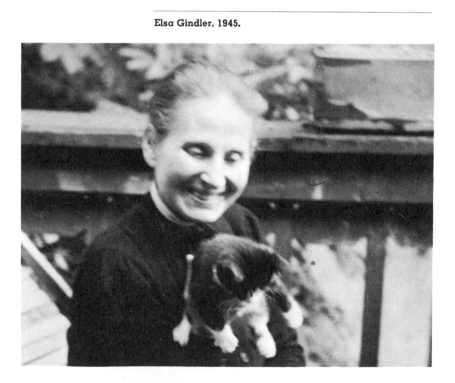

sense one's own functioning, and, beyond that, to sense and allow changes in the attitudes accompanying it, was not only possible, but could in fact become an approach to living entirely different from learning methods and practices handed down by others. What had at first been an intuitive therapeutic attempt became a *Weltanschauung* far beyond any bounds of therapy. Until her death in 1961, she pursued and explored this approach in practical experiments with many devoted students and without giving her work any more formal or specific name than *Arbeit am Menschen* (work on the human being) or *Nachentfaltung* (unfolding afterward).[1]

The last thirty years or so of Gindler's life were spent in intimate collaboration with another extraordinary pioneer in the processes of human learning and creativity named Heinrich Jacoby, whose classes in Zurich, exploring improvisation in music, acting, and the arts, finally became merged with hers in a long series of summer vacation courses in Switzerland. At the time I studied with him, in 1962, he had become mainly interested in education, and his class was full of young teachers from the public schools. Jacoby's conviction was that the way children spontaneously learn to talk was the prototype of all organic learning. Since this was hardly the method in the public schools, some of his students began to despair of their careers. Finally one asked him what she should do, since she now realized how unnatural, and even destructive, it was to teach as she would be obliged to. I shall never forget Jacoby's answer. "Why should you quit?" he said. "Someone less concerned will only take your place. Continue as you are, and don't

---

1. The utterly compassionate and realistic character of Gindler's attitude is evidenced by the fact that she not only continued to give her classes throughout the bombing of Berlin in World War II, but also gave special classes for her Jewish students, at the risk of being sent to a concentration camp if she were discovered. She even concealed a number of these students in her basement, feeding them with her own and her other students' scanty rations. By a tragic irony, a week before the arrival in Berlin of the Russian armies a Nazi youth flung a fire bomb into her building. The ensuing holocaust destroyed all of Gindler's records as well as the shelter of the Jewish students, who were promptly taken by the Nazis and killed. This, I have reason to believe, was the hardest blow of Gindler's life, far overshadowing the months of bombing, or her own early medical death sentence to tuberculosis.

worry about it. But there will be times, once in a while, when you instruct more than is truly required of you. Be alert for those times. Then, instead of the usual instructing, you can slip in a seed that will sprout into independent exploration." He died the next year.

Jacoby published one or two brief monographs.[2] Voluminous tapes of his classes are still in preparation for publication in Germany. It was his belief that there are no ungifted people.

Charlotte Selver was one of a few students who brought the Gindler work to the United States before World War II. Since 1938, Charlotte has been actively developing her approach to Gindler's work in this country. During the early years among new people with a new language, she finally settled on the now well-known expression "sensory awareness" to single out the awareness of *direct perception*, as distinguished from the intellectual or conventional awareness—the verbalized knowledge—that is still the almost exclusive aim of education, both in the family and in school.

Charlotte's work caught on very slowly. Her first advisers were agreed that Americans would never have the patience for it. But in the forties a number of New York psychoanalysts, most notably Erich Fromm, Clara Thompson, and Frederick Perls, became interested and began to study with her. Perls later incorporated much of what he discovered in his study of sensing into his Gestalt therapy. Then, in 1956, Charlotte Selver met the philosopher and Orientalist Alan Watts, who exclaimed as he worked with her, "But this is the living Zen!" Thereafter, the two collaborated in a long series of joint seminars, first in New York and then in California.

In 1963, introduced by Alan Watts, she gave the first experiential workshop at the newly founded Esalen Institute. This led swiftly to a wide dissemination of popularized and often misleading versions of the work throughout the country. "Sensory" interludes were soon being given to all the psychological and

2. Heinrich Jacoby, *Muss es Unmusikalische Geben?* (Zurich, 1925). Although Gindler and Jacoby assembled a great deal of material, almost none of it has been published. Most of Gindler's was destroyed in 1945, as mentioned above.

sociological discussion groups who assembled on that lovely ledge above the Pacific, and the fame of the relief from talking that was provided by these nonverbal experiences spread far and wide. This was also the year in which, after five years of study, I began to share the teaching.

In 1966 a collaboration was begun between Charlotte and me and the Zen Center in San Francisco, based on the experiential and nonconceptual elements which sensory awareness and Zen hold in common. This collaboration has augmented yearly.

The most recent development in the dissemination of this work was the setting up in 1970 of the Charlotte Selver Foundation, at 32 Cedars Road, Caldwell, New Jersey 07006, a nonprofit organization dedicated to the transcription of tapes, publication of bulletins and other literature, registry of sensory awareness teachers, possible establishment of a Center, and general furtherance of the work in the United States.

B NOTES ON ZEN

For the steadily diminishing number of people who as yet have not even an intellectual familiarity with Zen Buddhism, let alone an experience of the Zen practice of sitting called *zazen*, it may be helpful if I attempt to clarify the frequent references to Zen and *zazen* in this book.

There is a fascinating literature on Zen, which the interested reader may find in many libraries. It is the least intellectual and most experiential form of Buddhism, as it finally flowered in Japan. I, myself, have little scholarship in this field, and not a great deal of experience—merely a strong sense of kinship and respect. Many readers may know more of Buddhism than I, and a fair number will have had longer, or deeper, experience in *zazen*. My references are simply a consequence of this feeling of kinship, which has been reciprocated by many people involved in Zen practice. It is to clarify what is comprised in this kinship, and what may not be, that I wish, even at the risk of seeming presumptuous, to express myself on certain important and subtle matters.

Buddhism, in the West, has always been classified as one of the "world's great religions." It might thus be presumed to have a *creed*, as for instance Christianity does, and a cosmology, as all the religions do, including Hinduism. Its "Eightfold Path" might well be equated with Divine Commandments, its "meditation" with that in Christian retreats or in patristic theology, its forms and ceremonies with the symbolic rituals of Church, Synagogue, or Mosque.

Inasmuch as sensory awareness, as practiced by Charlotte Selver and myself, brings into question all established patterns both of gesture and of thought (whether established by gradual development in the culture, or by conditioning in the individual), it would be important, in this connection, to know if Zen does likewise. Also, since many insights and recognitions arising from our practice are of the character which has often been called "religious experience," it would be important to find what the word "religious" might mean to us. It is these questions which I hope a few words on my admittedly limited understanding of Zen may clarify.

To begin with, I should not hesitate to say that Zen Buddhism can no more be explained than life itself. There is no frame of reference that it fits into. But one can speak of a good many things which it is *not*.

Zen Buddhism is not a religion, as I would use the word. At least, as I understand it, it has no divinity or creed, and in the Christian sense neither revelation nor hierarchy. Nor is it a philosophy, in our traditional sense of systematizing experiences into a conceptual structure, or of organizing concepts into a system. But though neither philosophy nor religion (and neither physical nor metaphysical), it occupies the place in consciousness for its followers that these disciplines do for Westerners.

I would call Zen Buddhism an attitude, reached intuitively through example, intellectual self-discipline, and clearly recognized experience, nonverbally or semiverbally communicated, flowing easily into *relativity*, which to me is at basis no doctrine but a recognition.

Zen Buddhism has rituals, as sensory awareness does not, but rituals without symbolic value. Unlike the Eucharist, for example, the Japanese (or, for practical purposes, Zen) Tea Ceremony[1] has no significance beyond what is immediately expressed and perceived. It is fully in the here and now and has no reference to past or future or to other worlds. The Tea Master, being simply what Abraham Maslow might have called a "self-actualized" human being, must of necessity give far more of himself than need the priest, who can rely on a super-

1. Cf. page 123.

natural power delegated from "above," and as a person can be negligible.

Buddhist scriptures, also, are not "divine revelation" and do not function as the basis of faith in what has not been experienced. Buddhist vows are dedications, not the submission to a Lord's commands. Buddhist grace at meals gives acknowledgement for sustenance brought through "the labors of other people and the suffering of other forms of life," not thanks to the personal kindness of an "Almighty" who has placed all other beings at the service of man. In this absence of authoritarian structure, there could, I suppose, be no "psychology of Buddhism," as Freud's of Judaism and Christianity. On the contrary, psychologists are more and more turning to the study of Zen, not in order to explain it in their terms, but to help understand themselves it its terms.

There are sects in Zen, differing mainly in emphasis, and there is organization, so I suppose the word must be spelled with a capital. Existentialism, humanistic psychology, and sensory awareness, Western movements in this direction, can still be spelled without. But these movements lack the many centuries of human dedication which has developed the *form* of Zen—which Buddhist texts call the same as *emptiness*.

Zazen is the name for Zen Buddhist "meditation." But this choice of words may very easily lead to a misunderstanding, just as the reader may easily be a little puzzled by my use of the word "meditation" throughout this book. The traditional Western practice of meditation, as I think most of us understand it, has consisted in pondering the conceptual mysteries of "life" and "death," "good" and "evil," "God" and "man," et cetera, which at bottom, as the Greek root of the word "meditate" declares, means *thinking about* them. But *zazen* is the very opposite of this. Surely it would not have come to be called "meditation" at all were it not that the "meditative" man, in Western eyes, is he who has taken what seems the only alternative course to thought and action for worldly gain. Certainly the practice of *zazen* lays up no treasures on earth, even if the Chief of Police of Rangoon, as Admiral Shattock[2] writes, de-

2. Cf. page 47.

voted six weeks a year to the Burmese equivalent, while in the next cell was the owner of the local milk monopoly. Though it may be an unparalleled instrument for fuller living, as hinted by the *samurai* statement at the front of this book, it is still a full turning away from "practical" affairs. Its difference from Christian meditation lies partly in that it *seeks* no gain at all, either in this world or in any other. Thus it is equally a turning away from the prime considerations of our religions, which have always been how to find and obey the revealed will of an external God, and at some time in the future to be admitted to his heaven.

Zazen consists in sitting silent, motionless, and thoughtless on a small cushion on a mat for extended periods. One sits if possible in full or half-lotus position, or at least cross-legged or on one's calves, though this is not absolutely necessary. The eyes are partly open, but lowered, and though wide awake, and of course seeing, they do not look; neither, as often in yoga, are they controlled: only the impulse to wander is controlled. In the same way, motion is not controlled, but only the itch to move. Nor is thinking controlled, but only the compulsion to think.

Thus the organism is freed of its habitual drives to act, and is left available for perception. But for perception of what? It is not just the thought reflexes, and the muscle reflexes and observation, that are held at a minimum; it is reflexes from the whole sensory apparatus. If there is a sound, one does not listen; if a smell, one permits no association. Pain in the legs should not lead to judgment or to thought. Then what is perceived? Sensorily, everything; intellectually, nothing. What sounds is heard, but purely, for itself, as if it had never been before. Pain is experienced, but without anxiety or concern. If a recognition comes it comes, but it is not pondered.

But all this is not the "purpose" of *zazen*, which is stated as Enlightenment. This, like Zen itself, is *ipso facto* indefinable. I might think of it as the full experience of existing—which, strictly speaking, is a meaningless thing to say. It is significant, nevertheless, that a beginner is instructed to give full attention to his breathing (and in fact often to count it from one to ten), without allowing anything else, except his posture, to occupy his mind. In this case, obviously, all sense perceptions other than the proprioceptive and the sense of gravity are distractions. No one expects the beginner to be free of them, but his *attention is to be directed* only to his sitting and his breathing. Such attention is central, if not exclusive, in our work also.

All over the world, I suppose, breathing is associated with the central fact, or essence, of living—as in such words as *spirit, animate* or *animal, breath of life, last breath.* It also represents our most regular and intimate relationship to our environment; and its uninhibited functioning involves more of our flexibility and musculature than any other organismic activity. Finally, it is the only major such activity governed equally by the voluntary and involuntary nervous systems.

The concern with breathing in *zazen* is not for the purpose of improving it, but simply that one may become more and more conscious in connection with it. Of course, such consciousness can easily become "self-consciousness," which always entails a split in the personality and an involuntary self-control. But in *zazen*, just as in the practice of sensory awareness, one may feel after a while that one is not so much conscious *of* breathing as conscious *in* breathing. One becomes identified with breathing and no longer an observer of it. Then whatever becomes conscious as an inhibition of breathing becomes an inhibition of oneself, whether it is a force from the "outside" or from the "inside": self-consciousness, self-observation, introspection become a restriction, just as a halter might. More, it is not a restriction of *oneself*; it is a restriction of life. One is no longer divided between oneself and the other, between observer and observed; self-criticism—in fact, any criticism— is no longer possible. It is not even *one's* breathing: one *is* breathing. Breathing is what one is.

But breathing does not occur in a vacuum; it requires air, just as it requires a living organism. Breathing is not the air, nor is it the organism: it is the interaction between them. If one *is* breathing, one is interaction. One is somehow both the inside and the outside.

As theory this need not concern us. But as experience, it could illuminate for us the actions of those Buddhist protesters in Vietnam who burned themselves alive, perhaps because they felt the reality outside them as more than equal to their own self-sacrifice, and who may have taken this ultimate step in reaction to a *recognition* rather than under pressure from an Idea. It could also illuminate the attribute of Buddha as the Compassionate One, and the strange-sounding Buddhist vow to save all sentient beings. The difference between one who looks to a Savior for such a purpose and one who vows it himself must be the difference between one who maintains the division between himself and others and the one who feels the division can be given up. The meaning of saving all sentient beings can be only the feeling that between all sentient beings and oneself there is no real boundary.

But this statement could not be made at all in a Judaeo-Christian context of absolutes. As in the recognition of Einstein, it would be the relativity and interrelationship of everything that alone had significance.

So it may be understood why I have a semantic objection to the term "religious" as qualification for those deeper and seemingly truer experiences which artists, poets, musicians, dancers, and lovers have shared in common with many historically "religious" people, and with many who patiently followed any form of meditation, and which may also be the fruit of the patient and loving practice of sensory awareness. This is a practice which gradually sheds belief, symbol, and symbolic ritual, leaving us, as does Zen, free of rewards and punishments, prayers and judgments, hopes and regrets, fully in the here and now.

C REPORTS

The following are included because the direct and vivid quality of the writing seems to me to make a valuable addition to what has already been written.

A (*A psychologist and group leader*) In one of the first sessions, Charlotte spent over an hour with us working on what appears on the surface to be a very simple thing: one member of a pair simply lifts the other member's hand and then returns it to rest. But as Charlotte worked with us, and with mild suggestions gently led us to strip away all kinds of activity unrelated to the pure task of lifting the hand and letting it down again, there came to be a kind of clarity in my experiencing of myself. I found myself able to give up all the other kinds of associative activity and unrelated muscular activity and simply allow my hand to be lifted or to lift my partner's hand. I was led to give up concern about the partner: I gave up feeling close or distant, or attracted or repelled; I gave up being reminded of other times when my hand was lifted or I lifted another person's hand; I gave up sexual connotations of the touch; I gave up concern as to whether I was holding my body right; I did nothing other than allow my hand to be lifted, and then later to lift my partner's hand. And in that moment of clarity, I think I experienced what Charlotte means by "being fully present for what you're doing" and I got some glimpse of the wonder of being able to live so that one is fully present for whatever is going on. There was an incredible clarity to the event, a startling simplicity in just allowing the other to lift my hand or allowing myself to lift my partner's hand; but at the same time, there was the recognition of an immensely full and complex process which is ordinarily obscured and confused by the process of association, of muscular holding, of trying to attribute meanings and intentions and transferred emotions to that specific concrete situation that really have no business there.

For a brief time during that experiment, I was a whole being, functioning in a holistic manner. I was no longer mind carried by body. The experience was illuminating. I was also in no way beclouding the existential event of having my hand lifted, by expectations from the past, or plans for the future. I was simply being in the present, and I experienced a burst of energy, of great heightening of awareness and an excitation of creativity in those few minutes that I recognized from previous times but the nature of which I had not understood so clearly before. There were many other experiments that weekend but that particular one stands out as a kind of moment of understanding which is in no way intellectual and which is so badly communicated by intellectualizations. (S.K.)

B *(A photographer)* One day you asked us to go down and come up again, to squat. I didn't know what to do; I was almost petrified. This was something I had not been able to do in years. I knew I would fall over, or have to go down on all fours to get myself up again. But, gritting my teeth and holding my breath, I did it—down and up as fast as I could. I didn't go down very far, but I went down and got up again without falling over. How did it happen?

We did it again and again. Each time I dared to go a little farther down, a little more slowly. Strangely, the slower I went, the more easily and smoothly. I began to feel the change of balance in my torso, the bending in my hips and knees, the tightening of the muscles in my thighs. It was still frightening and a little painful, but how exciting! To actually squat down and come up again—something my head had told me I couldn't do; and I couldn't do it before, not until I stopped listening to my head and let the whole body take over its normal functions. Much later I discovered that I could also kneel and sit back on my heels, something that had previously been agony to me.

After many experiments, I began to realize that my immobility was the result of fear-constricted muscles, which in turn constricted breathing and circulation. There was fear of falling, fear of pain, fear of failure and ignominy, and these fear-constrictions were holding tight all the muscles that had to give for mobility. These realizations came in the muscles themselves, in those occasional experiments where this holding was given up and I could move freely, with a blissful feeling of well-being.

Parallel to these realizations about the "inner world" came the understanding that when these inhibiting muscle/breathing/circulation-constrictions could be given up, there resulted a more open relationship to the "outer world" as well. Naturally, these newly rediscovered abilities to kneel and squat were the greatest delight to me in gardening, where I had formerly grunted and groaned in getting up and down, and suffered considerable backache and often nausea from hanging over with all the organs scrunched up in the middle of me. (Experiments in hanging made me recognize this fact, and learn how good it feels to hang from the hip joints, with plenty of room in the torso for breathing and circulation.) Now I enjoyed getting up and down. It was wonderful to experience the feeling of strength and ease as I moved, and I gave myself plenty of time to appreciate it.

I found that, in being open and unhurried to the delicate changes within me, I was beginning to be open and unhurried in my relationships to everything around me. I was able to recognize the differences in the weeds I was removing, and respond accordingly: to allow time to follow a long, brittle stem of the chickweed through the grass to the small, clutching root, pull it out, and lift the long tangle of stems without breaking them; to pull out the long, heavy root of the dandelion in just the right direction and with just the strong, steady pull needed to get it out without breaking off a piece to send up another plant; to get just the right hold on a clump of slippery wire-grass to be able to pull out its big clump of roots. And to be able to do this without damaging the flowering plants the weeds were crowding out. None of this was intellectual; it was purely sensory awareness.

In like manner, I was able to be more considerate of plants I was putting in the ground, observing at exactly what depth they needed to go; that they were not too crowded for their future size; that they would get the amount of light they needed. And I was more open to the beauty of form and texture, light and shade—the fragrance of the flowers, the foliage, and the earth.

So where does it end? Does it end? As I became better able to sense and respond to the plants according to their needs, I became better able to listen and respond to my children, my friends, anyone.

As you said, after we had squatted and come up again, "It feels good, yes?" Yes. (M.A.R.)

        C *(A professor of medicine)* I'm sure you must be fully aware of how much your Tassajara workshop meant to me. The beauty of the experience must have been written all over my face, my bearing, my very being. But I really want to put down in writing some of the feelings which emerged.

I have always come naturally to being sensorially aware. As a child, I would like to blur my vision and watch the abstract forms and lights dancing on water, or listen to night sounds, or smell old houses, or whatever. But you opened up unimagined vistas. Instead of asking myself, what can I see, what can I hear, what can I smell, I am now open to the experience of experiencing, whatever the experience may be—within myself, the natural world external to myself, or my relations with other persons. I have a long way to go, of course, as mindless,[1] untrained, unlearned, unprogramed experiencing is such a

1. I believe the word "mindless" could here be considered the exact equivalent of the *mindfulness* of page 47—i.e., full attention without intellectual activity. This points up the great difficulties we so often come into when we use those many words (usually ones we value highly) as to whose precise meaning there is little real agreement. Such words can only be read intuitively, in a context. [Author's note.]

new idea to me that I have just begun to open up to this whole new exploration. However, this is as nothing compared to the awesome discovery, while passing the ball back and forth from my hands to my partner's hands,[2] what it really means to give, to receive—without a contract, no negotiation, no expectations, no past, no future—just giving, just receiving. What flows? What is it like? What happens? . . . Fifty-three years I have lived, and I don't think I ever received anything from another human being, that is, was not able within myself to receive—simply, fully, gracefully, gratefully—until about six months ago; but the full impact of this marvelous capacity of one human being to give to another human being, and to receive from him, did not get to me until passing the ball. Suddenly I found myself literally transported into another world of being. The tears flowed. I was a little self-conscious, although not embarrassed. Or, better expressed, it was an intensely lyrical moment for me; it was personal, and I did not want to be on display. I sat quietly in back, hoping no one would notice. Suddenly I was aware that J—— S—— was next to me, quietly, her fingertips just touching my arm, just to say that she was there if I needed her, and I pushed my head hard into her lap so that I could sob convulsively without making a sound, and I could share this moment with J—— only. But, of course, I want to share it with you, as you brought it about, and it expressed, more than any words I could write, what had happened to me during the beautiful week of the workshop, culminating in that magical moment. (A.B.)

2. See pages 199–200.